HOLDING TIME

HUMAN NEED AND RELATIONSHIPS IN DEMENTIA CARE

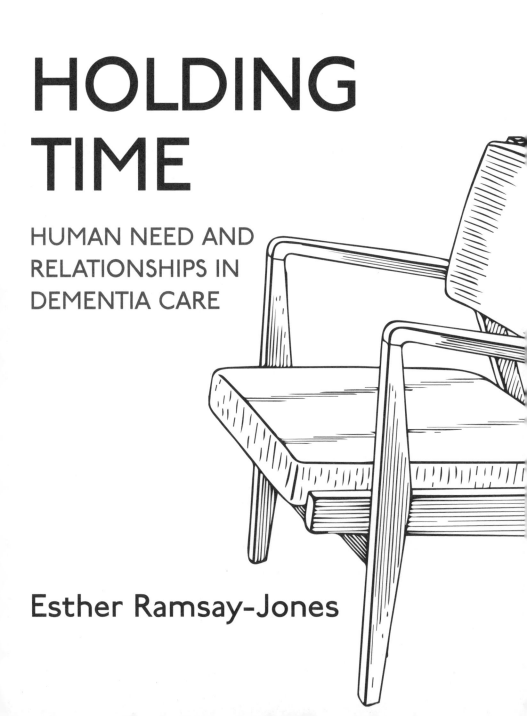

Esther Ramsay-Jones

First published in 2019 by
Free Association Books

Copyright © 2019 Esther Ramsay-Jones

A CIP Catalogue of this book is available from
the British Library

ISBN: 978-1-91138-325-3

Typeset by
Typo•glyphix
www.typoglyphix.co.uk

Cover design by
Candescent

Chair illustration from
Pixabay.com

Printed in the UK

I don't know what to say
Yep
I'm making a statement.

The Things Between Us, Living Words: Anthology 1.
Words of people experiencing dementia. (2014, p. 150)

TABLE OF CONTENTS

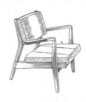

ACKNOWLEDGEMENTS

I wish to thank the older people in residential care homes with whom I have worked and who have over time taught me so much about meanings in human life. There are too many to name here, who have shared their insights and discomforts and humour, and who have fired up something deeply existential in me. Specifically, meeting with Daphne and Dorothy has been a great privilege, even though it was at times painful to endure. I also want to thank Melie who, in my previous incarnation as a care worker, eased me into the role playfully, with her ability to continue to give, despite her confusion and wordlessness. My gratitude extends to all the carers who allowed me into their worlds, many openly, despite some fears that I may have been a critical figure representative of the intensified surveillance in the working context. I found myself often hanging on their words, knowing sometimes that people were sharing stories that had not had an outlet before. I hope on those occasions that I listened well enough.

Thank you to Dr Gail Lewis and Dr Peter Redman for sharing their experience, ideas, thoughts, and approaches, and taking a much-needed critical stance at crucial moments; to my lovely family, Matt, Eloise and Fearghas, who have supported this endeavour all along the way, with mischievous grounding interruptions! And to my Mum and Dad, who in their older age show our small family what it means to sustain a caring relationship.

INTRODUCTION

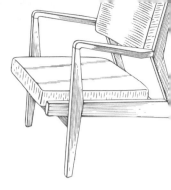

I go total blank… trying to work out what it's like without the… most of the pieces aren't here so I can't put names to them. And we're dropping downhill slightly. I planted these up but I can't remember now what we are really looking at… and some of them are growing very well… that's lovely. Some are not so good because they are not in a good place. And I start asking where I live and where I am and so on and I can't tell you now, let alone then. I can't… I've forgotten about it all and why… I don't feel I was together at all and my hair's all over my eyes which is driving me crackers.

Ellen, Whittinghall Care Home

The seed of this book was sown over a decade ago when I started work as a carer in a residential care home for older people in London. People had warned me that it would be hard work, and that I was over-qualified. My husband feared the work would be demeaning, as if it were also a narcissistic blow to our combined sense of self, and our aspirations for the future. There was, and perhaps still is, a sense of shame that surrounds care work with older people with dementia (Clough, 2016). It is viewed as low-status and carers are heard to describe themselves and their colleagues as 'arse-wipers' (Jervis, 2001, p. 89). As Clough (2016, p.33) points out, 'In a culture where money determines value, many care workers feel grossly undervalued' and, she goes on to write, quoting Sander et al (2011),

As a society, we displace our discomfort with human frailty by removing it to hospitals and care homes, packaging it with targets that attempt to regulate and sanitise it and creating a culture of shame when these targets cannot be met.

(Clough, 2016, p. 33)

Back in 2003, I did not reflect long on issues of institutional shame. I was also unaware that people with dementia in care homes, and their carers, could be split off from the rest of the wage-earning community, ghettoised in groups of failing populations. Nonetheless, I must have been unconsciously drawn to this hidden old age and to death and to experiences which would often escape words, try as you might to pin them down.

Certain memories come to mind when I ask myself what drew me to care work for older people: me as a pre-pubescent child, noting my insignificance in relation to the full expanse of the planet and knowing that one day I would die; a neighbour in her seventies, who called me in from our street for lemon and honey tea, garishly dressed, recounting stories from her days as a fashion buyer; my grandmother, Faith[1], who, with Alzheimer's, maintained a belief in both people and God, which seemed to help her to settle into a care home in Wales, easing her journey into death. Somehow, both these older women seemed to come to accept the expunging of breath and of existence – my greatest fear. Perhaps for existential reasons I have needed to get closer to decline, dependency, and death in order to know more about how any of us, as temporal beings, become reconciled with our own finitude.

Choosing to work with people with dementia, in particular, relates consciously to my grandmother's experience, and to the experience of confused voices and voicelessness. Here, one of my prime concerns has been to find ways to make known those voices that either struggle to articulate in language their own experience or those who – like professional carers – are left silenced because society undermines their contributions, which cannot often be monetised. The experience of newborns, for me, is a powerful evocation of the need to make feelings known: the baffling cries of my own babies; my newborn self even, outside the order of words, a new Mum, anaesthetised, tired and in pain, her baby behind an incubator without her; Dad anxious and alone. And there back home, the newborn screaming, legs up to chest contorted in colicky distress and parents rocking and rocking and rocking her. All of these unknowns and imaginings play out when I begin to think about my reasons for entering the field of dementia care, leading me to ask questions of self and others, and of what it is to care, how hard it can be to do so.

---

1 All names and identifying features have been anonymised.

Yet questions about what constituted professional dementia care only really began to emerge when I met Melie. Melie had thick white curled hair and it stayed on her head precariously like billowing candyfloss. She had her own teeth still but they were yellowing and cracked and uneven. She had small eyes that squinted and didn't let much light in until, that is, we started to play and Melie burst into life with me. I was her keyworker, one of the first people I had ever keyworked. I felt unknowing and amateur, but with Melie I knew that we worked together. We would often walk around the home, making mischief. She would hide behind curtains and pop out, a glint of knowing in her eyes followed by lots of deep and meaningful laughter. For want of a better word, I thought that I loved Melie as a friend, as someone I cared for, as a surrogate grandmother, who knows? But I looked forward to work because I looked forward to seeing Melie.

Looking back on the work I did with Melie reminds me now of a scene in May Sarton's (1973) *As We Are Now*, a beautifully nuanced account of being abandoned in a care home, narrated by Caro Spencer, a seventy-six-year-old former teacher:

> *Sometimes Anna can sit down for a minute after my breakfast... She is not a talker. I feel perfectly at peace when she is there and we do not need words. She seems to understand me in a way I have needed for years... it is being cared for as though I were worthy of care. It is being not humiliated but treasured.*
>
> (p. 92)

Melie and I were perhaps more playful than Caro and Anna, but we were open to one another; quite possibly we had to be because Melie had lost all capacity to speak. She articulated sounds, walked, ate, she could even dress the bottom half of her body. But speech had gone. So we created a new language that moved around between us through bodily mirroring, eye contact and plain noticing. We noticed the other, each other, and did a dance in which both selves could take turns.

Melie could never say she wanted to go to the toilet and so she rocked, her torso reaching out into the room and her bottom half rubbing up against the cushioned sofas. Over time, I knew what this meant, and others did too. She could see when I got tired and sometimes her hand would reach out to my cheek, as if she knew that I had had a busy day.

Of course, this kind of gentleness (sometimes seen as sentimentality) doesn't always sit well in what can be a brutally task-driven institutional environment where jobs have to be done, and timetables have to be adhered to. In fact, not all interactions with Melie were gentle. This kind of relating changed into something altogether more confrontational when it came to cleaning Melie's teeth. The intrusion of an object into her mouth – the mouth that could no longer speak – infuriated her. She would bite down on the toothbrush, shake her head, check her rage out in the bedroom mirror, and sometimes scream 'No', the only word she had kept hold of. You learned to go slower at tooth-cleaning time. You learned to offer Melie the brush, letting her assess it. Sometimes you would take the brush yourself and play at brushing your own teeth. Sometimes this worked; sometimes it didn't. And what you began to ask was, given Melie was in her late eighties, what shame was there in her failing to brush her teeth? There was more shame in her going to sleep unsettled with clean teeth whose shininess had been forced upon her.

This time with Melie taught me about relating outside the order and structure of language, and it conveyed something profoundly human. You could see her desire for continued connection, for play, for struggle, for agency, for dependency, interdependency and independence. When I became a mother, the spectre of Melie was around. This is not to say that she was a pre-verbal newborn baby, a toddler or a child, but it is to say that that these very human needs, so visible in babyhood, manage to last with us, I think, to our dying days.

This book is an investigation into the experiences of seemingly voiceless people, who can be spoken for and about without reference to the complexity of their experience. It is also about mapping, describing and analysing the relational field in dementia care, exploring what facilitates and prevents connection. It is also about mothering, understood in its broadest sense, the kind of mothering that involves reflecting on raw, sometimes unprocessed experiences that belong to individuals and organisations, working out how they may link, and finally reframing them – with the help of psychoanalytic theory – so that they may make a little more sense. By telling the story of two residential care homes, through the observations of older people, Dorothy and Daphne, and through interviews with staff and other residents, I hope to be able to say something about working and living in a care home and about the importance of these experiences. I want to consider what both helps and hinders 'going-on-being' (Winnicott, 1960) and working in such environments. How do groups of humans continue to demonstrate concern for one another when some practices and policies seem designed to thwart this aim?

The Socio-Political Background

There are 800,000 people in the UK living with dementia. The King's Fund (2008, cited on Alzheimer's Society online, n.d.) projects the financial cost of dementia to reach £34.8 billion per annum by 2026, a 135 per cent increase from 2007[2]. In April 2012 the World Health Organisation pushed for dementia to become a global world health priority. *The Guardian's* Haroon Siddique (2016) published statistics showing that Alzheimer's disease and other dementias have now replaced ischaemic heart disease as the leading cause of death in England and Wales for the first time.

In terms of policy, the seventeen recommendations in *Living Well with Dementia: A National Dementia Strategy* (DoH, 2009) emphasise better care in care homes and improved staff training. The first *Prime Minister's Challenge on Dementia* (DoH, 2012) claimed that 'Health and Care' would be one of its main areas for action. In April 2013, NICE launched a new set of quality standards on care, 'Supporting People to Live Well with Dementia' (NICE, 2013). The *Prime Minister's Challenge on Dementia for 2020* (DoH, 2015) highlighted the importance of care home research. Developments such as these place the question of dementia care and the quality of the caring relationship high on the agenda of policy makers. Or at least this is how it seems.

In recent years, however, social care in England and Wales has been increasingly subject to cuts, austerity and neoliberal reform[3]. As the Alzheimer's Society points out:

> *Dementia care and social care are, largely, the same thing. Where other conditions need medication or devices to alleviate symptoms, the symptoms*

---

2 The number of new cases are 40,000 fewer than previously predicted (Matthews, FE et al., 2016).

3 Reporting in *The Guardian*, Butler (2016, n.p.) writes: 'Government cuts have resulted in a £4.6bn reduction in social care budgets in England since 2011, representing a real-terms net budget cut of 31%.'

of dementia affect people's ability to do day-to-day things – washing, dressing, eating. With no cure on the horizon and few treatments, people with dementia are relying heavily on care to meet the basic needs caused by the symptoms of their disease. Social care is the only treatment they have for their disease. Further to this, people with dementia are the majority of people receiving that care – they make up over half of people receiving care from paid carers in their homes, and are nearly three quarters of people in care homes.

(2017, n.p.)

Recent reports also demonstrate that the care sector is routinely undervalued. Quoted in *The Guardian*, John Kennedy claims that:

managers are finding the role almost untenable as the complexity of their job grows and they face an external regulatory system increasingly adversarial and critical… they feel vulnerable and alone. The role of registered manager is a challenging one. Even a small care home will have a turnover in the millions, a significant workforce and more rules and regulators than you'd care to count. Even so typically salary levels are only in the mid £30k range. No other sector bestows so much responsibility on its management cohort with so little recognition or reward.

(Sodha, 2016, n.p.)

Managers are under ongoing strain and we know that there is endemic abuse of the minimum wage laws in the care sector:

Data from the Office for National Statistics showed that between April and June this year [2016], about 113,000 of the 769,000 workers who provided at-home care for vulnerable people or were employed in care homes were on contracts with no guaranteed hours. At approximately one in seven, that total represents a substantial and rapid increase on 2015, when one in ten care workers were on zero-hours deals.

(Osborne and Duncan, 2016, n.p.)

Lay (2017) reports that social care cuts were linked to 30,000 excess deaths in England and Wales in 2015, based on findings from research conducted by the University of Oxford in collaboration with London School of Hygiene and Tropical Medicine and Darwen Borough Council.

Professor Martin McKee, from the London School of Hygiene and Tropical Medicine, stated:

> The impact of cuts resulting from the imposition of austerity on the NHS has been profound. Expenditure has failed to keep pace with demand and the situation has been exacerbated by dramatic reductions in the welfare budget of £16.7 billion and in social care spending. With an aging population, the NHS is ever more dependent on a well-functioning social care system. The possibility that the cuts to health and social care are implicated in almost 30,000 excess deaths is one that needs further exploration.
>
> (University of Oxford, 2017, n.p.)

Politicians' statements and media reporting often collude to suggest there is an ageing population at bursting point, generating huge costs to our economic systems. A leaked memo from then Pensions Minister, Baroness Altmann, which was reported in *The Guardian*, talked of the 'looming crisis [of social care] which has been left far too long already', and pointed out that the government has not done enough to avert the 'potential social and economic distress' (Boffey, 2016, n.p). Her memo suggested that older people start to set up care-ISAs for their impending social care costs, since local authorities had no money set aside for the demographic changes. Similarly, in 2013, Jeremy Hunt advised families to take in their loved ones in later life (Butler, 2013, n.p.). However, Manthorpe and Illiffe (2016, p. 14) claim there is a 'high level of societal anxiety about dementia... [which] stems from the myth that an ageing population causes the costs of health care to rise dramatically'.

Appleby, Chief Economist at The King's Fund, points out that the projected costs of a growing ageing population has been exaggerated:

> The ageing of the population is also a factor, although of much less importance than is generally supposed: increases in life expectancy tend simply to delay the time at which the health care costs associated with death are incurred rather than increasing these costs per se. This is an important point as it challenges the conventional thinking that spending on health care will rise inexorably as the population ages. In fact, the pressure to spend more will largely be driven by other factors.
>
> (2013, p. ix)

He claims that long-term economic projections are riddled with uncertainty. To date such increases relate mainly to investments in technical and medicinal innovations, not necessarily in direct care.

Apocalyptic visions of an ageing population at bursting point (eg, the paralysing image of bed-blocking), are presented in policy and in the national media. It is as if there has been a move to stir up fear, and possibly hatred, of ageing populations – symbolising in the unconscious mind a drain on resources[4]. The metaphors and stories associated with dementia are often accusatory, persecutory. These narratives merge together, blindsiding the public, and perhaps preventing it recognising that austerity measures and the adoption of a managerialist approach to welfare lead to failings in the social care sector.

Relatedly, there are 'new consumer expectations about better managing long-term and immediate care needs' (Manthorpe and Iliffe, 2016, p. 14). However, with rising expectations, resources for health and social care have been systematically cut.

The gap between the expectation and the reality of service provision arguably creates a sense of deprivation. A consumer narrative within policy has partly fuelled this widespread sense of inadequate service provision, which appears all the more inadequate when spending isn't forthcoming. There are, simultaneously, real and entrenched inequalities. The crisis is felt by all those no longer able to access services but in a sense the crisis is also exaggerated. This exaggeration relates to the managerial restructuring of welfare systems (Froggett, 2012) in which the consumer/ service user is increasingly set up, intentionally or not, to demand more in terms of targets, timescales and outcomes. On a psychic level, people start to feel deprived by the parental figures of government, which may mean that splitting, rivalry, and abuse become par for the course in the public rhetoric around ageing. All of this is the result of a long-term strategy, embarked upon in the days of Thatcherism, to shift radically the terms of sociality in which the ethic of care for the 'stranger' is stripped away (Hughes & Lewis, 1998; Lousada & Cooper, 2005; Layton, 2014; Hunter, 2015).

In the care field similar mechanisms might be at work. The care home, after all, is a society, on a micro scale. We have heard of abuse

4 A split representation of ageing: 'active ageing' versus failure narratives. Available at http://apps.who.int/iris/bitstream/10665/67215/1/WHO_NMH_NPH_02.8.pdf

in residential care homes. A series of high-profile cases have drawn our attention to what goes on when there are systemic organisational failings, where we might surmise marginalised staff members in turn brutalise marginalised residents – the latter raging against the former for reminding them of their own fragility, powerlessness. To name a few, we have Hillcroft Nursing Home in Lancashire where residents were used for staff entertainment (BBC Online, 2014); hidden cameras at the Old Deanery in Essex where staffing levels were 'woefully inadequate' (Dugan, 2014) and abuse ensued; Purbeck Care Home in Dorset where cruelty and neglect were widespread (BBC Online, 2015); Keldgate Manor Residential Home where Freda Johnson, eighty-five, suffered regularly at the hands of the staff; and BBC *Panorama's* (2016) account of a nursing home run by the Morleigh Group where a resident was left for forty minutes stuck to a bedpan, where morphine was used as a patient cosh.

What I hope to consider in the unfolding of this book is how intimate, meaningful relating nonetheless remains a possibility in an overarching socio-political context which attempts, purposefully or not, to destabilise, or denigrate, our connection with one another on a basic human plane in favour of a politics of self, of individual success (Layton, 2014). When dementia care policies weave together voices from activism, advocacy and psychology with those from the markets, big business and advertising, which voice is in the end the most powerful? What is the small daily revolution that allows people to show concern and make contact in an economically driven care marketplace?

We have a crisis in social care and health care, where the cutting of resources leads to inadequate staffing. Paradoxically, the quality of the caring relationship and a responsive 'workforce' is still a government expectation. What quality means within such relationships is rarely defined, and care workers are asked to do something increasingly difficult: to be compassionate with little compassion afforded to them; to be compassionate without time or space to reflect upon what this means, to process the difficulties raised by the work.

Manthorpe and Iliffe (2016) make the important suggestion that the government's over-focus on medical care and scientific research needs refreshing, and an approach that is 'relational rather than technical' (p. 14) needs greater investment.

The Caring Relationship

Thinking about the relational, which Manthorpe and Illiffe (2016) highlight as an important omission in *Living Well: A National Dementia Strategy*, is fundamental. The complexities of the professional dementia care relationship are manifold. Often, there is a disconnect between the ways in which the carer and the person with dementia experience time and their immediate environment. A professional carer of someone with dementia relates daily to a person who is experiencing the gradual dispossession of mind (Dartington, 2010), yet the emotional labour of the caring work frequently goes unrecognised.

It is this question of the quality of the caring relationship in a residential care setting that is at the core of this book. It was from the notion of maternal subjectivity, and a sense that it might have some useful applications to the field of dementia care, that this exploration was born. Maternal subjectivity is defined in relation to an-other, the infant, and vice versa: the relational is arguably written into the experience of mothering practice. As Donald Winnicott noted:

> *There is no such thing as a baby... If you set out to describe a baby, you will find you are describing a baby and someone. A baby cannot exist alone, but is essentially part of a relationship.*
>
> (Winnicott [1946] 2017, p. 98)

It was my experience as a mother which reawakened my thinking about dementia care. When I held my second newborn and he cried, sometimes raging for milk, I began to think about pre- and then post-verbal experiences. The feeling of dread when we imagine that there is no one there to gather us up; of fragmenting into different pieces of existence with no recourse to being put back together; hungry in the belly and hungry in the heart. I started reflecting about myself, as a mother and earlier as a carer. What did this intense encounter with dependency stir up in me? I wondered what the post-verbal adult, unbecoming in his dementia, stirred up in the worker, expected to comfort and contain?

However, a person with dementia is in no way a newborn. Firstly, someone with dementia is moving in the opposite direction of becoming; people with dementia have had lives and experiences that newborns have not yet encountered. Memory traces, from womb to old age, make us who we are and so, even when factual detail fails us, we continue to carry within some memory of being elsewhere. A person with dementia has known herself perhaps as a boss, an employee, mother, father, brother, sister, schoolchild; as stubborn, intelligent, joyful, antagonistic, warm. These knowledges of self don't shed themselves completely as dementia takes hold; a person with dementia remains, often holding on tightly and simultaneously slipping away. She remains in the sense that she meets with the world in familiar ways; tries to preserve whatever agency she has had as much as she can; wishes to be treated with a degree of respect as someone who has participated in the lives of others. Within her, she also carries the newborn, as we all do, and possibly the fears and desires of dependency and connection. What then goes on between the recipient and provider of care? *Holding Time* examines whether organisations have a way of supporting both the desires and fears of dependency/inter-dependency that seem to me to be written into humanity, our need to be *with* and to be supported by others while also wishing sometimes to be alone. It seeks to understand how organisations deal with the experience of being cared for: what it is like to be looked after by another person and therefore vulnerable to him or her, however careful he or she is. How is expression given to this experience in a professional dementia care context?

The Chapters

Relationality in Dementia Care begins with a theoretical account of the mother–infant dyad and how the figure of the mother and infant are constituted in psychoanalytical literature. The representation of mothers found in psychoanalytical literature is not idealised but is, instead, textured, multi-layered and attuned to the emotional realities involved in the work of mothering. This chapter focuses on the mechanisms that underpin the affective flows that take place between both parties and demonstrate, where possible, how psychoanalytic ideas can provide further insights into ideas about relationality in dementia care discourse (Kitwood, 1997; Miesen, 1999; Browne & Shlosberg, 2005; Adams & Gardiner, 2005). This focus on mothering, which is not to detract from the importance of fathers too in the development of children, is tied into the recognition that in our earliest experience of dependency – in utero and just after birth – we are developing in relationship with a mother's body and mother's mind. In dementia, we are returning to a state of increasing dependency and perhaps it is this relationship with a mother figure that is most often evoked, on a deeply psychic level.

The chapter adopts a theoretically pluralistic approach, drawing on Melanie Klein (1930; 1937; 1952a; 1952b; 1952c), Donald Winnicott (1946; 1953; 1958; 1960; 1962; 1971), who developed contrasting clinical paradigms, and post-Kleinian, Wilfred Bion (1959; 1961; 1962a; 1962b). The relational psychoanalyst, Jessica Benjamin's (2006; 2007; 2010) work on mutual recognition is also important in this field, as is Lacanian psychoanalyst Bracha Ettinger's (2006; 2009; 2010) radical exploration of subjectivity. Her structure of the developing mind takes in networks of multiple subjectivities and traces of human relationships, even in utero, which offer an exciting way of making sense of the patchwork of dead and existing identities found in dementia care.

The processes involved in mother–infant relating that seem pertinent to the dementia care field in particular include projection and introjection, containment, holding, and play. The second part of the chapter focuses on psycho-spatial concepts, such as the organisation-in-the-mind (Armstrong, 2005) that explore the dynamics and tensions in organisational life and the capacity to engage with care work in general.

Winston Grove and *Whittinghall* will introduce both care homes, and most importantly Daphne and Dorothy. The aim is to give the reader a sense of what it was like *to be there* in the homes, as a resident, as a worker and as a visitor. As such the passages set the scene in everyday language that seeks to convey the emotional texture of life in the homes without interruption from theory. Stepping into the shoes of Daphne and Dorothy and feeling their way around the care home environment as they do is the aim of these chapters. They are based on a series of ongoing psychoanalytically informed observations. Though this work involved a rigorous ethical review with the awarding body, I have also altered the material in order to anonymise the experience of the older people and professionals with whom I spoke, producing in many ways a piece of writing that intersects with psychoanalytic, ethnographic, and literary genres.

The following chapter *Time* hears from residents and staff in Winston Grove and Whittinghall, in their own words, reflecting upon what hinders and what supports human connection. As per the observations, many details have been changed and, owing to issues of capacity, I sought consent on a frequent basis throughout. The understanding of time is nuanced, multi-layered. Residents and staff understand its conceptualisation differently. Time is a major preoccupation in care homes with older people with dementia, and the aim here is to unpack its meaning using psychoanalytical thinking. In essence, the chapter considers how time can be used most appropriately to provide good care to both residents and staff.

Mothers abound in the care home environment, figments of imagination, figures of projection and sites of repair. Mothers are simultaneously absent and present, calls for mothers and for home permeating day-to-day life. This chapter endeavours to make sense of the different qualities of mothers that emerge both in the lives and minds of residents, and in the staff team, particularly when the latter discuss their reasons for doing the work.

Culturally in the West we may be entering a time of death revival (Clarke, 2018), but in the care home sector a silence often surrounds death. *Death* presents a discussion about the difficulty of working in the face of death, and the defensive strategies employed to cope with, or to deny, this reality. This chapter examines the difference in approaches between both care home sites, and points to the learning that can be drawn from both. The learning from each thematic chapter is enhanced by drawing on psychoanalytical theory. However, the socio-spatial context in which dementia care is offered is not forgotten. Woven throughout each chapter is a recognition of the neoliberal frame, and the general push towards new managerialism and the under-resourcing of services. There is some discussion of experiences which are often felt to be inarticulable in the care home environment, such as class and race, and yet which enter into the relational field, affecting human dynamics.

Finally, the book ends with a conclusion about the lives of Daphne and Dorothy, as well as some thoughts about the current national policy domain and a personal reflection on the strange uncomfortableness society experiences in the face of other people's dependencies – and hence our own.

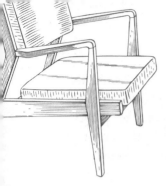

RELATIONALITY IN
DEMENTIA CARE

Care of the very elderly, those so often lacking the capacity to speak, yet so intensely riven by extreme emotional states, requires a painful reversal of the original pattern of container/contained (very often the young now struggling to offer states of reverie to the old).

Margot Waddell, *Inside Lives: Psychoanalysis and the Growth of the Personality* (2002, p. 249)

Introduction

This book is heavily indebted to psychoanalytical thinking, drawing on various traditions (object relations, the Independent School and relational psychoanalysis[5]). The theoretical frame for this exploration is a pluralistic one and, though the history of psychoanalysis has, at times, been riddled with 'unhelpful splitting and polarised' rivalries (Keane, 2012), different aspects of psychoanalytic theory apply to the experience of being in both care homes as cared-for, or as worker, and to the emotional atmosphere of care settings.

Borden (1998), struck by the way in which Winnicott guarded against the compulsion to make things known, writes:

---

5 This work uses object relations theory in relation predominantly to Melanie Klein's work. Although she noted the developmental significance of the primary relationship, her work arguably over-emphasises internal mental states and perhaps the noisier bodily drives, such as hunger. The Independent School, also known as the Middle Group (used interchangeably here), is considered post-Kleinian object relations in its focus. This group highlighted interpersonal context, often observing real relationships, as seen in the work of Winnicott and Fairbairn, and possibly the quieter drives for soothing, holding, very much dependent on object-relating.

Winnicott, ever concerned about the dangers of omniscience, works to undermine 'the impression that there is a jigsaw of which all the pieces exist'... More than any other figure in the Middle Group, Winnicott comes to emphasize the crucial functions of missing pieces, gaps, the "spaces between," and the areas of unknowing in our use of theory in practice.

(p. 37)

Borden suggests that others, such as Bollas, have also attempted to work in a way supportive of theoretical pluralism:

Each Freudian should also be a potential Kohutian, Kleinian, Winnicottian, Lacanian, and Bionian, as each of these schools reflects a certain limited perspective.

(Bollas, 1989, p. 99, cited in Borden, p. 33).

This idea of drawing from multiple theoretical frames is inspiring. The psychosocial milieu is one which conjures up notions of multiples in the sense that it is not a one-theory approach, not least because psychosocial endeavours try to create a bridge between two worlds – the psychic and social – which have been presented and treated by the division in academic disciplines[6] as if they are fundamentally different. Sociology and psychology attempt to capture aspects of human experience, and then proceed as if distinct. A psychosocial approach begins with the premise that the psychic and social are not distinct but are rather ways of seeing and understanding experience, which can be in conversation together.

Furthermore, the experience of dementia is full of moments of not-knowing. Valerie Sinason (1992) writes of her work with a client with dementia:

From knowing, possessing knowledge, words, thoughts, there is a downward path towards not knowing. It means returning to the first chaos of infancy when not an infant and having possessed knowledge at its fullest and finest.

(p. 89)

---

6 'Social' being the domain of sociology and 'psychic' as the domain of psychology.

Using a range of theories is a reflection of my own not-knowing and the not-knowing involved in the work. Approaching the stories and words of the residents and staff in both care homes presents a counterpoint to the push – in current policy and practice – to get it right and to make certain the uncertain.

A pluralistic approach resonates with the work of David Armstrong (2005), whose concept of the organisation-in-the-mind is a useful place to start. In *Organisation-in-the-Mind* (Armstrong, 2005), it is clear that his model of understanding organisational cultures draws from the theories of Klein, Bion, from clinical psychoanalysis, as well as organisational consultancy. Some suggest (Hutton, Bazalgette & Reed, 1997) that the organisation-in-the-mind is a Winnicottian transitional object, which offers possibilities of understanding a client's relatedness to an organisation through his *me* experiences in role and the *not-me* experiences of the consultant attending to the material.

The psychic life of the individual and the organisation are at the heart of this investigation and, as a result, drawing from theories which are one-body, and which emphasise interior space, and those which deal with the intersubjective realm, are both important. The following quote from Armstrong (2005) relates to both dimensions.

> *Every organisation is an emotional place. It is an emotional place because it is a human invention, serving human purposes and dependent on human beings to function. And human beings are emotional animals: subject to anger, fear, surprise and disgust, happiness or joy, ease and dis-ease.*
>
> *By the same token, organisations are interpersonal places and so necessarily arouse those more complex emotional constellations that shadow all interpersonal relations: love and hate, envy and gratitude, shame and guilt, contempt and pride – the several notes of Joyce's 'chambermade [sic] music' – a wonderfully apt phrase for the emotional choreography each of us weaves, consciously or unconsciously from our encounter with another, or with others.*
>
> (p. 91)

Of course, dementia care takes place in an intersubjective space and you will see that the nature of the carer (the external object) had implications for the psychic sustenance of the person with dementia. However, instinctual drives, particularly anxieties around living and dying, were often expelled into the care home atmosphere, and were – in a classically Freudian way – possibly related to the biological/neurological changes that people with dementia were experiencing.

This chapter demonstrates how psychoanalytical ideas can provide a richer account of human behaviours in the context of dementia care than perhaps general dementia care literature. The latter has nonetheless offered an intuitive understanding of the person with dementia, from which some very important innovations have emerged, but psychoanalytical understanding perhaps takes us further.

Psychoanalytic thinking concerns the psychic development of the subject, from birth onwards. The experience of dementia is possibly a reversal of the developmental trajectory of the infant, from dependence through to relative independence: how, then, does psychoanalytical thinking help us to understand this reversal?

GENERAL THEMES

The literature on relationality in dementia care involves the following concepts, all of which provide some understanding of the (inter-) subjective experience: personhood, attachment, recognition, mirroring, embodiment, ethics, and the senses. The number of writings on relationality is growing and emerges from a variety of disciplines, from social psychology and psycho-gerontology to nursing and the behavioural sciences. Some, like Pia Kontos (2005; 2014; 2017), draw on philosophy, sociology, and the arts. Those writing on attachment-seeking behaviours and parent fixation in people with dementia, in which a mother or father is believed to be alive (Miesen, 1993; 1999; Browne & Shlosberg, 2005), are inspired by the work of Ainsworth (1978) and Bowlby's influential work on attachment patterns in children (1979). Paul Terry (2003; 2010), a clinical psychologist and psychotherapist, and Tim Dartington (2010), a former researcher from the Tavistock Institute of Human Relations, draw predominantly from psychodynamic theory and the lived experience, as do Balfour (2006) and Davenhill et al; Davenhill (2003; 2007) . Others (Adams, 2005; Ryan et al, 2008; Nolan et al, 2004; Ellis & Astell, 2010) conduct practice-based research to formulate frameworks to help those working as nurses or carers. Much of this work has led to an exchange of important ideas, as well as some shifts in approaches to frontline care work and in national policy.

Many improvements in the field can be attributed to the work of psycho-gerontologist Tom Kitwood (1997). His work had a long-term, positive impact on dementia care practice; his focus was on the subjective experience of someone with dementia. Kitwood pioneered a person-centred approach in dementia care. One of his (1997) achievements was the development of Dementia Care Mapping, a practical tool used to isolate and identify harmful behaviours found in staff teams working with people with dementia.

The term 'malignant social psychology' (Kitwood, 1997, p. 48–49) was coined by Kitwood to describe the collective impact of a pervasive set of behaviours among staff teams in dementia care institutions that damaged the care recipient's sense of self, personhood. These included objectification, infantilisation, invalidation, and disempowerment (Kitwood, 1997, p. 47). Although Kitwood's work has been foundational to improvements in dementia care, he does not explain how malignant social psychology might emerge. In line with Menzies-Lyth's (1959) contributions, it is possible to argue that psychoanalytic theory provides such an explanation, as well as further understanding about the intersubjective processes which lead to poor care. In deploying psychoanalytic theory, this book will endeavour to explain, at least in part, how such a malignancy might emerge.

In terms of ethics, Millet (2011) applied embodiment discourses and bio-phenomenological ideas to the concept of self and dementia. He argues that a person with dementia, although struggling cognitively, remains a being embedded in the social world, able to affect those around him. Quoting Jonas (1984), Millet (2011) says: 'The newborn is the perfect paradigm, literally the prototype, of an object of responsibility' (p. 518); her mere existence places a demand on us. For Millet someone with dementia, like the newborn, is particularly vulnerable to harm from the world and there is an ethical imperative to care for and to relate to her.

At this stage, we might turn to babies in psychoanalytic literature. We know there are different types of babies in psychoanalytic theory, though always assumed to be an object of responsibility. What differs among theorists is whether the baby is fundamentally pleasure-seeking (pain-ridding) or object-seeking from birth. We might argue that the Kleinian baby is generally considered insatiable, riven with destructive impulses. For Klein, these destructive, or envious, impulses are rooted in the death drive, considered innate to human experience. The energy of the death drive needs to be bound with the forces of the life drive in order to mitigate internal conflict and tension. It is up to the mother to rid the baby of these kinds of frightening bodily discomforts, returning through her milk the experience of pleasure. Winnicott's baby is also hungry, but his primary motivation is to form primary affectional bonds. A Winnicottian baby also displays aggression but this stems from frustration, when response from the primary carer is not forthcoming. For him, early object relations can produce gratifications leading to an internal state of tranquillity. This is not just a modification of painful states.

For clarity, there was a major difference between Freudian and Kleinian schools of thought and later Independent traditions. As Keane (2012) points out, there was a paradigmatic shift from Freud's biologically determined theories based on drives and their transformations, over development, to an increasing emphasis on the structural changes in the personality which resulted from internalised object relations that took place externally. Klein fell somewhere between the two. She didn't relinquish the fundamental drives of life and death, yet acknowledged that object relations are there from birth. Apart from the drive/object emphasis, a further distinction between Kleinian and Winnicottian theory relates to the assumption about the degree to which there is an ego that is to some extent integrated. In line with Winnicott's interpersonal emphasis, Winnicott implies that ego integration is a developmental achievement, supported by holding, maternal adaptation, and so forth. Klein says less on this subject, but proceeds as if there is an infant that has some level of integration, an ego which often finds itself split.

The point of convergence, however – despite the difference in emphasis between ego integration or not, drives versus object-relating, or mother as shadowy external figure, simply modifying intolerable experiences in the infant, or mother as an object of attachment – is that the mother figure is nonetheless assumed to be responsible for the infant and for the development of his sense of self, his ego strength. The mother–infant relationship is fundamentally asymmetrical, which is also generally true of the relationship between carer and cared-for.

Benjamin's (2009; 2018) baby is also part of an asymmetrical relationship. However, this baby is beginning the process of weaning, an older baby. He has an increased sense of agency and independence. Benjamin's theory of mutual recognition and thirdness revolves around the increasing separation of mother and baby. Finally, there is Ettinger's

(2006; 2009; 2010) foetus. Unlike other theorists, Ettinger highlights womb existence. Ettinger's foetus is always-already an agential subject. This seems vital for dementia care because Ettinger assumes that all human beings, from conception to death, are both agential and social, collaborative. In dementia care, then, when people with the condition might be thought to be lacking in cognitive function and capacity, there are ways in which individuals are well able to express their own needs and, when facilitated by an intimately understanding relationship, those 'voices' are well able to be heard.

Resonant of Ettinger, Millet (2011), indebted to Levinas, claims that there is an a priori ethical responsibility towards others which hinges on the fact that human subjective life is socially embedded from birth. Millet counters Davis's (2004, in Millet, 2011) claim that dementia leads to 'the very splintering of the sedimented layers of Being' in which the 'life-world dissolves into background meaninglessness' (p. 518). For Millet, people with dementia need not experience a social death. Psychoanalytical theory – particularly the work of Bion and Winnicott – helps us to understand the interactional processes which might lead to one party experiencing a social death. Here, Bion's (1962b) notion of 'nameless dread' and Winnicott's (1960) 'going-on-being' seem particularly evocative. These forms of psychic dying are related to two different sorts of caring (maternal) failures. For Bion (1962b) the experience of nameless dread comes about in relation to the mother's failure to make meaning out of an infant's projections of existential fear; for Winnicott (1960), the interruption of being takes place in the context of a mother whose holding, both in mind and in arms, function is shaky.

Returning to dementia care, Ellis & Astell (2010) developed an intervention, Intense Interaction Therapy, in order to sustain someone's personhood, to avoid a social death. This intervention involves interacting with people with dementia, often with those who are post-verbal. The therapy involves validating and mirroring the communications of the person with dementia. Ellis & Astell (2010) found that people with dementia had rich communicative repertoires that used sound and signal. This became richer when a carer reflected back the sounds and gestures of the person with dementia. Although vital work, it does not detail the dynamic psychic processes encountered during such communications – communications that Klein (1946), Bion (1962b), and Winnicott (1960) so eloquently describe throughout their work.

The psychoanalytic understanding of the mechanisms through which people engage and disengage with one another would, arguably, benefit much of the dementia care literature. Adams & Gardiner (2005) situate their work on dementia care triads alongside those who have critiqued Tom Kitwood's (1997) person-centred care for failing to 'fully capture the interdependencies and reciprocities that underpin caring relationships' (Adams & Gardiner, 2005, p. 186, citing Nolan et al, 2002, p. 203). They see their work as offering a fuller picture of care exchanges and aim to minimise the polarised and polarising experiences of informal carers, people with dementia, and professionals by paying closer attention to subjective experience. However, like many others adopting a relationship-centred approach (Nolan et al, 2004), the recommendations that stem from the research are often abstract.

Nolan et al (2004) argue that 'person-centred care, as defined in the National Service Framework, is not the panacea that it is held up to be' (p. 46). They make a convincing case for 'valuing interdependence' (p. 47). Ryan et al (2008) point out that relationships are fundamental to good care, suggesting that six particular senses underpin good relationships for people with dementia and staff: a sense of security, sense of continuity, sense of belonging, sense of purpose, sense of achievement, and sense of significance (p. 80). These are important aims, yet the research has omitted to consider how complicated processes of relatedness can be; and the six senses seem to be conceptualised as static once achieved, as if states of mind are never in flux.

Dartington's (2010) exploration of Alzheimer's disease is based on his wife Anna's early (fifty-two years old) onset experience of dementia. He offers an insight into dementia that is personal, political, and psychoanalytical. He touches on the theme of recognition, writing: 'It is our sense of our own self that is affronted. And we act as if the other has lost his identity, is not the person he was – a perception that is as true (or false) about ourselves as it is of him' (p. 151). Dartington rages against a journalist's lack of compassion when the writer claims that people with dementia are stripped of their 'memory, their personality and eventually their humanity' (p. 193). He is reminded, in the bleakest of times, of his wife's humanity when she laughs at the Queen's broadcast on Christmas Day. 'What, he asks, are the "clinical signs of loss of humanity?"' (p. 193). As we are increasingly aware, people with dementia might be in a state of cognitive decline, yet there is an ongoing, and complex, emotional awareness (Balfour, 2006; Dartington, 2010; Davenhill et al/Davenhill, 2003, 2007) that may be conveyed in stories, memories, and bodily and unconscious expression. As Balfour (2006) poignantly asks, 'What might remain, at an unconscious level, of the experiences of people with dementia, whether or not they are consciously able to articulate them?' (p. 332).

The way in which we construct ourselves in relation to others is as much a concern for dementia care as it is in infant care. Although someone with dementia might appear to be slipping away, advocates of good practice in dementia care suggest that the person continues to exist but in changing forms. Frazer, Odeboyde and Cleary's (2012) discussion of women with dementia who live alone highlights an interesting phenomenon. The women in their study, at least in the earlier stages, started asserting their identity as a past-life, at times forgetting themselves in the present. Frazer et al (2012) argue that *now* signifies incompetence and losses beyond comprehension. A return to earlier stages of personal history represents earlier competencies, a time which feels more recognisable perhaps. Recognising someone with dementia involves recognition of him in the present moment, of what is being lost and of the bewilderment that dementia entails, as well as the earlier selves that might come to inhabit him. In this context, Winnicott's (1971) theories of play might be helpful, particularly in facilitating the possibility for someone with dementia to re-experience himself, or to experience himself, unjudged, anew.

Tim Dartington suggests that someone with dementia might use forgetfulness defensively, in order to split off depressing realities of change. He references music therapist Davenhill (2007, cited in Dartington, 2010, p. 151), who talks about the ego emptying itself out, as a way of understanding the emotional and physical deterioration in dementia. This psychoanalytic lens, based on Kleinian ideas, provides us with a way of thinking about how the person with dementia no longer seems the person we once knew. Dartington argues that without recognising these processes, it is possible that a mutually defensive interactive style, an avoidance of each other's pain, begins between carer and cared-for whereby neither is recognisable to the other.

Kitwood undoubtedly felt it was imperative to reclaim personhood for someone with dementia, whereas others have wanted to acknowledge explicitly the importance of relationships in effective care. I hope that a psychoanalytic reading will be able to provide a further dimension to understanding the care relationship, the shifting subjectivities, the development and un-development of mind, which Dartington (2010) and Terry (2003; 2010) point towards.

In 'My Unfaithful Brain', Anna Dartington writes about her experience with a plethora of different carers. With one carer, she might have an experience of her 'choices becoming less' her own (Dartington, 2010, p. 158), but with another she will have negotiated the world on her 'own terms' (p. 158), and found in a carer a new 'mother' (p. 158) able to inspire in her a more bearable mode of being.

It is interesting that Dartington speaks of carers as mothers because psychoanalytic theory assumes that the mother–infant dyad[7] – notably from Klein onwards – is the foundation stone for all future relationships. (We might be reminded of Miesen's (1999) work on parent fixation in which a person with dementia, moving further towards dependent states of being and the intolerable experience of organic and emotional losses, might increasingly call out for a parental figure in order to manage his or her fears.)

What, however, psychoanalysis might offer, which other theorists working on relationality in dementia care only hint at, is an understanding of the processes and mechanisms involved in such intimate relating. Psychoanalytic ideas help to disentangle what we imagine about other people (how we construct them in our minds) from what might belong to us; how we transform others as much as they transform us. As Redman's (2005) examination of transference and countertransference demonstrates, many psychoanalytic concepts also arguably provide 'an inherently relational understanding of the unconscious dimensions of affective experience' (p. 52).

Mother–infant relationships

ETTINGER: THE MATRIXIAL

I will start with Ettinger (2006), a Lacanian analyst whose work is at the intersection of clinical, maternal, and artistic experience. What is striking

---

7   Freud's tendency was to avoid situating the regulation of inner tension in an interpersonal context (ie, with mother/or father). Secondarily, fathers, grandparents, professional caregivers can also take on the role of primary caregiver in an infant's life.

about Ettinger's work is its focuses on the growing foetus and woman growing into mother. It teeters on the philosophical in the sense that, at base, a reliance on another is part of the originary make-up of human beings. Ettinger captures a primordial experience, less reliant on the notion of mental development than the other psychoanalytical thinkers. Her work resonates with aspects of dementia care, particularly because this can be a post-verbal time, where communications are embodied, and also a time of profound dependence.

Ettinger's background is Lacanian, yet her interest lies in the pre-Imaginary and pre-Symbolic experience, the pre- or trans-verbal of the infant subject. For Lacan, language determined the order of the subject, enveloping him/her in a series of symbolic associations and signifiers. Human subjects 'model their very being on the signifying chain that runs through them' (Lacan, 1956, p. 21). Relating, at a conscious level, is made available through language, yet language also creates a distance between people. The process of intersubjectivity – and subjectivity itself – is an alienating one in which everyone is bound by the order of the signifier and signified.

Ettinger, though, is concerned with an experience that precedes language, which does not alienate. For her, there is an inarticulable residue of human experience which grounds us as subjects. This experience is always related to the site of the mother, a wombspace which leaves unconscious pre-verbal memory traces – an asymmetrical residing-in another, (m)other. The notion of asymmetry is also relevant for dementia care, since relating at this stage of life might stir up memories of asymmetries that characterised our earliest experiences, good and bad. Balfour (2006), writing specifically on the experience of dementia, indeed notes,

'At the other end of life… we see how there can be a breaking through of earlier unresolved emotional constellations, appearing now as phantoms in the mind, the return of the long-ago ghosts of the nursery.'

(p. 335)

For Ettinger, the foetus, relying on the ebb and flow of nourishment, via the umbilical cord, is a symbol of our originary experience of dependence, and of care. The baby is not without agency, however, as any mother would testify when she sees the outline of legs protrude from her extending stomach with each kick. Written into human experience is the sharing of bodies, psychic spaces, a pre-verbal co-existence between two subjectivities-in-becoming who call the other into being (Ettinger, 2009, p.13).

Mother and foetus relate to one another in a sub-symbolic co-emerging, which Ettinger describes as trans-subjectivity (Ettinger, 2006, p219). The mother, in connection with the growing infant, distances herself from assumed earlier senses of self. Changes taking place in the growing foetus have an effect on the bodily and emotional experience of the mother.

Ettinger describes momentary encounters between two beings-in-becoming who experience in one another, at the deepest unconscious level, a simultaneous difference and sameness in a shared space. We might be reminded of Winnicott's (1971) concepts of *me* and *not-me*. In Ettinger this holding-in-tension of neither subject nor object is experienced in the womb. This is interesting because this capacity to be neither fully 'I' nor 'you' has resonances with Winnicott's sense of potentiality. In other words, perhaps our truest self involves an openness to experience, one which doesn't foreclose on thinking by categorising being and identity into either *me* or *not-me*, a state of being that is not entrapped 'behind' hard (defensive) boundaries. There is an openness in this, which at the best of times might be seen in professional care when moments of co-affecting take place.

As Hollway (2011) highlights, the founding image of a life growing within a life-in-change is an experience that pushes at the 'boundaries of available language' (p. 24). Ettinger develops a new vocabulary in which concepts belong to a careful balancing of difference and sameness, which she demonstrates in her use of hyphenation (for example, 'differentiating-in-jointness'; 'encounter-eventing'). This hyphenation reflects her belief that the human subject is simultaneously touched by others and yet separate. Hers is an ontological language that resists splitting and makes space for collaborative contacts. Her subject is not alienated, tentatively moving towards and away from objects; rather her subject is implicitly capable of existing alongside other subjects and objects simultaneously.

This has resonance with Kristeva (1985), when she points to a form of maternal love, which gives the 'speaking subject... refuge when his symbolic carapace shatters to reveal that jagged crest where biology transposes speech: moments of illness, of sexual intellectual passion, even death' (p. 152). Kristeva reminds us that language acts for the speaking subject as a protective shell, an armour, out of which we construct notions of ourselves; that via language we engage with others as subjects who are never fully articulated. Kristeva speaks of the unconscious language of biology – an existential trace that rests in the body's earliest experiences – which perhaps links to moments of the newborn's handling. It is the maternal that Kristeva summons up, comforting in times of discomfort, sexual union and even death. This takes us to the bewildering experience of dementia, where the symbolic often fails and when people are in need of solace, of a presence, sometimes outside language.

The feminine-matrixial resists both the narcissistic self (I/self), constituted through the language of self and object, and the forces of endless fragmentation experienced in a fused oceanic state (Ettinger, 2010, p. 2).

It is worth noting that Ettinger seems to be interested in borderspaces. Professional care work is very hard, and from my observations it also seemed very precarious, both psychically and in political reality. It was tempting for care workers to make their world feel more certain by polarising experiences and by applying neat categories and divisions to things and people. Ettinger might point to the usefulness of being able to encounter in one's experience chaos and order simultaneously (the order of a bounded identity; the chaos of feeling what others feel).

In good circumstances the maternal subject in Ettinger neither returns to a fictitious autonomous pre-child self (Baraitser, 2009), nor does she lose herself completely to the infant. Rather she allows herself to self-fragilise (Ettinger, 2009). It is this idea of the self-fragilising mother which may act as a useful paradigm for all the caring professions: a process of opening up to the disturbances, joys, pains of the 'client' without entirely fragmenting in relation to another's emotional realities. A professional able to self-fragilise is thus one who would not resort to rigid defensive modes (Menzies-Lyth, 1959) of functioning, neither would she be incapacitated by empathy. Encountering another person in this way in daily care work would most likely require a good deal of organisational support.

From this vantage point, Pollock (2008, p. 10, cited in Hollway, 2011) argues that the matrixial lays foundations 'for our capacities for ethics, hospitality and compassion for the other in their otherness' (p. 13) while also having a level of thoughtful compassion for ourselves.

Although Ettinger's conception of the matrixial is grounded in a time in utero, her work has some links to Winnicott. Ettinger's matrixial thinking is complementary to Winnicott's concept of primary maternal preoccupation (Winnicott, 1958). He describes an infantile experience before a singular stratum of individuality is acquired and when the infant needs an extension of the 'compassionate hospitality of the womb' (Hollway, 2011, p. 34).

Winnicott claimed that in the weeks after the birth, many mothers experience an unsettling mental state. The mother is closely attuned to the needs of her infant by creating a near-perfect fit between demand and response. In this short time her infant's demands take up the central place in her body and mind. Again the notion of asymmetry in the relational encounter is in play. If we are to apply this to Ellis & Astell's (2010) research, mentioned earlier, we might expect the professional carer to make the effort to contact the person with dementia so that communication between the pair becomes possible. The carer brings the person with dementia to life, like Winnicott's (1958) adapting good enough mother.

Winnicott (1962) used the word 'matrix' – the Latin word for womb – in his paper, 'On the Capacity to be Alone'. Ogden (1990) teases out the meaning of the term matrix in Winnicott's paper as the 'silently active containing space in which psychological and bodily experience occur' (p.180). Ogden is describing what Winnicott termed holding. For Winnicott, the infant's psychological matrix is the maternal holding environment, and he views the infant as being highly sensitive to any changes in this environment. This holding environment provides a near perfect adaptation to the infant's changing emotional and physical needs, but also to maturational ones. Winnicott's matrix, resonant of Ettinger's matrixial, has a womblike quality but is now external to the mother's body. It is the responsive adaptation to the infant that provides this sense of continued wombspace, of holding. Arguably, holding facilitates the experience of going-on-being, which in turn relates to a developing sense of self embodied in space and time. Holding is an important function in good dementia care, where a person may be calling out for continued being in the context of a shaky temporal and spatial frame.

Holding involves a process of highly responsive micro-interactions to ensure that the baby feels in control, omnipotent. He is fed when hungry, touched when isolated, warmed when cold – all of these sensitive moments prevent the baby from falling apart in panic, as if he is not surviving. This survival depends in part on his being in the mind of someone else. This is the complex work of being held in mind (thought of) and handled (practices of touch, feeding) that go into forming the earliest structures of mind: 'yes, I exist'. Mother does this until the infant has developed his own internal psychological matrix, after which point the mother begins the process of weaning the infant from this consistent good-enough maternal provision of holding, handling and object-presenting. In dementia care, we are not talking about a movement towards integration, but rather the creation of momentary experiences of reintegration through holding. It is possible that Ellis & Astell's (2010) Intense Interaction Therapy might provide the kind of illusion of oneness that helps someone with dementia to continue to exist in the social world.

Winnicott's (1971) ideas on play are also helpful. Play is something that takes place between people, particularly small children and parents. Play creates a space (between the borders of individuals) in which nuance can be tolerated, where the conscious and unconscious sit hand in hand. Winnicott referred to 'potential space'. This is an intermediate area of experiencing that lies between the inner world and external reality (Winnicott, 1971, p. 55). In the early stages of development the good enough mother helps to create in conjunction with the infant a potential space in which transitional objects (Winnicott, 1953) are used to quell the anxiety of disillusionment; the realisation that mother and child are separate subjects and not fused. Transitional phenomena, dolls and soft toys, can be brought to life by the child, acting and talking with them, investing them with certain qualities of me and not-me. (Relatedly, Stephens et al (2012) conducted a systematic investigation into the use of physical objects by people with dementia, discovering that people with dementia can and do use objects in a way akin to the Winnicottian concept of the transitional object.) Any potential space is filled with the child's imagination, stemming from his internal experiences. Play is not judged in a good-enough playful context, which helps the child to be in touch with parts of himself that are spontaneous, creative and, for Winnicott, authentic.

In play, the child achieves a sense of self and autonomy, watching her internal world outside in potential space, while also negating 'the idea of a space of separation' (Winnicott 1971, p. 110) from her mother. There is a greater sense of self yet a continued connection with mother.

Play provides an experience of passage, a bridge, between separation and unity, a jointness-in-differentiation that is crucial to making meaning as an individual, who exists alongside others.

BENJAMIN: RECOGNITION

If we are to think of different psychoanalytic theories as dealing with different points on the developmental trajectory, we might think of Winnicott dealing with birth to weaning. Jessica Benjamin's (2006; 2009; 2018) theory of mutual recognition, facilitated by the opening up of a Third, focuses on an infant's journey towards greater independence and separateness from mother. The mother, in Benjamin's work, begins to take leave of her infant and disclose her separate sense of identity. This marks the time when a possibility opens up for greater degrees of symmetry (or perhaps more accurately greater degrees of being seen and of seeing). She says:

> *Mother, of course, ideally holds this awareness in mind from the beginning. But as time goes on each does something different to make it work. Mother is primarily responsible for making it work, for scaffolding the baby's action, while baby 'plays along.' The differentiating Third refers to an awareness of the distinct part played by the other required for the coordination and resonance to work, the 'something more' than just us two matching even while we are feeling 'at one'. This surplus attention to the other's regulation based on recognition of difference characterises the mother's asymmetrical responsibility.*
>
> (Benjamin, 2018, p. 82)

Jessica Benjamin's (1995; 2006; 2009; 2010; 2018) work on recognition has implications for dementia care. Benjamin argues that the process of recognition is central to intersubjective relating, in which both parties experience the other as whole, complex, and separate beings. In dementia care the person with dementia will need much more from his carer than he is able to give back. Recognition permits us to engage realistically, and altruistically, with one another, as whole objects, which involves inequalities, as well as equalities, sameness, and difference. In other words, an ethics of care involves the recognition that humans share in existential experiences of dependency, interdependency and independence but that there are numerous individual differences in our abilities to care at different times across the lifespan.

Benjamin (2006; 2009; 2018) offers us a hopeful picture of the relational field, in which seeing, noticing, recognising acts as a counterpoint to entrenched power dynamics between people. Benjamin's theory provides us with a way of understanding how we can go beyond a sort of narcissistic part-object form of relating, often at the basis of racism, sexism, ageism, for instance. As Benjamin (2018) points out,

> *Recognition involves knowing and being known, as in 'moments of meeting' when, as Sander puts it, 'one individual comes to savour the wholeness of another'.*
> (Sander, 2008, p. 169, cited in Benjamin, p. 77)

Neither party is therefore under the other's imagined, and omnipotent, control. Winnicott's ideas on play, where the parts of the self can be expressed freely and without fear, has some resonance here, too.

A process of differentiation is key to the production of subjective meaning for Benjamin (1995). The subject here is conceptualised as one able to manage difference and space in the context of a relationship. Benjamin takes a Winnicottian stance in so far as she believes that the infant's capacity for empathy grows out of recognising that the very person upon whom he depends is not under his omnipotent control. The mother's departure from her infant signifies a crucial learning experience – thus reminding us of Bion's (1962b) claim that we learn through a manageable level of frustration.

Recognition, from the perspective of the infant, is quite complex – he recognises Mother's separate subjectivity through Mother's absences, and sees that this symbolises his limited sphere of influence over her. The infant also learns that Mother also chooses to be there with him when she stays. Though the relationship – like an analytical one – is based on a form of 'asymmetrical responsibility' (Benjamin, 2010 p. 245), infant observation studies also demonstrate that the infant is able to communicate and make his desires known. What Benjamin describes is the possibility for greater symmetry embedded in a fundamentally asymmetrical caring relationship. I am reminded of the field of dementia care here. Although carers are ultimately responsible for residents' well-being, people with dementia do at times recognise the needs of a carer and help out in whatever way they can. As Ettinger (2006) might argue, at base we all have the capacity to be collaborative.

In the interactions that Benjamin describes, both parties make self-disclosures. Intersubjectivity occurs when such self-disclosures are recognised, rather than distorted through the lens of narcissistic desire, allowing for genuine contact to be made. Contact like this is considered a 'shared third' – both subjects have come to recognise interactively the other's subjectivity. The 'shared third' (Benjamin, 2009, p. 443) is a concept that has vividly spatial connotations. This space provides the opportunity for each party to recognise difference and connection simultaneously. Arguably, this notion of mutual recognition (Benjamin, 2006; 2018) offers a more relational view of care and has the potential to be a guiding idea for the helping professions.

The logic of much of Benjamin's work is that the infant's capacity for recognising the distinct subjectivity of his mother emerges through a process of spatial and temporal distancing – there is a paradox here in that psychic closeness (understanding that others have separate minds to respect) is achieved through greater distances of a spatial and temporal nature. However, someone with dementia may find it hard to recognise a professional carer in this way, not least because increased withdrawal of care staff (breaks, absenteeism) is likely to lead to further disintegration in someone with dementia. Breaks and endings in this context, as with the mother–child relationship, must be managed with sensitivity and care.

Ettinger's work on the matrixial, wherein the womb represents in our primordial unconscious the feeling of deepest security, and Winnicott's notion of primary maternal preoccupation resonate here. Only from a place such as this one – in which space and time is shared, rather than fought over – can we gather ourselves up confidently enough to claim a space of our own. It is perhaps as true in organisations as it is in the family that a process of sharing and joint-meaning making is needed before we are able to recognise divergent approaches, roles, and identities.

KLEIN: SPLITTING

This inquiry into the relational field of dementia care would have been lacking without Kleinian (1930; 1946; 1952a; 1952b; 1952c) object relations theory. Klein often deals with the destructive feelings involved in the emergence of human subjectivity. One of Klein's main assumptions is that the internal world of the infant is in conflict. The infant has tremendous difficulty in integrating innate anxieties about surviving. The Kleinian infant is one that tends to expel, or project, the bad stuff – rage, greed, hatred – and, all being well, Mother returns something better for the infant to introject. If Mother fails, then her dysregulation under the pressure of the baby's destructiveness becomes internalised as a broken self, the infant either identifying with the mother's collapsed state, or identifying with his own destructiveness. The external world becomes a precarious one, full of confused meanings.

A similar process might take place between a carer and a person with dementia. The cared-for, by the very nature of the condition, may already be in touch with her own internal precariousness each time she notices the loss of a word, a memory, a thing, and, fearing breakdown, may project this outwards into the environment. In turn carers may become receptacles for destructive, angry feelings. In essence, perhaps, an infant and a person with dementia might, at times of heightened primordial anxiety about survival, be calling out for rescue. In that moment, at a deeply ontological level, the infant or older person is in contact with the sheer intensity of human dependence. Undoubtedly, then, when the calls for help are met with silence, raging distress is inevitably expelled.

Although 'the struggle between the life and death instincts emanates from the id [forcing the ego into action]... the primary cause of anxiety, the fear of annihilation, of death' (Klein, 1952a, p. 57) exists in the infant at birth, coming from within, and it is through identificatory processes with the mother that subjectivity is gradually structured and, in good circumstances, shaped to become less split. The tensions between the powerfully incompatible drives of life and death begin to lessen once introjections of a good object begin. A shift to a more ambivalent position – a fusion between life and death – allows for the management of the drives. A responsive carer able to think about the projections of a person with dementia might similarly be able to minimise conflicts in the person she cares for.

In Klein, the source of the ego is tied into the instinct for life and survival, the need to feel integrated; the id associated with the death drive and (aggressive) libidinal force. As she points out,

> Opposed to the drive toward integration and yet alternating with it, there are splitting processes which, together with introjection and projection, represent some of the most fundamental early mechanisms.
>
> (Klein, 1952a, p. 57)

By projecting the instinct to survive outwards, 'by turning outward libido and aggression and imbuing the object with them, the infant's first object-relation comes about' (Klein, 1952a, p. 58). Through the process of introjection this object[8] becomes internalised. I am suggesting that processes of projection and introjection are taking place inter-subjectively between carers and people with dementia on a daily – and intense – level.

Like a dementia care worker, the mother, in Klein, is often under pressure to respond to violent projections. Although we have not come to him yet, it is important to point out that the mechanisms of projection and introjection were grounding ideas for Bion's (1962a) theory of the container-contained. Bion details the function of the mother more comprehensively than Klein did, though he built his theory upon these Kleinian mechanisms. Contrary to Winnicott, projection – the projection into – implies that there is never a period of a fused infant-mother pair in the work of Klein or Bion.

Klein's work does not present us with the hopeful, creative narrative of Ettinger's co-constructed emerging or with the ostensibly more gentle theorising of Winnicott. Klein shows us that the process of coming into being can be fraught relationally, and we might surmise that, for many with dementia, the process of leaving existence, the relinquishing of self, is also unbearable, catastrophic. From Klein's work, we imagine just how hard it can be to mother a baby. Extrapolating from this, and applying it to dementia care, we might also acknowledge how hard care work can be. After all, this is a job which involves responding to those who might be experiencing a deep, persecutory anxiety akin to the dependent infant's fear of dying.

There is conflict in the interplay between the real mother and child, as there might be between the person with dementia and her professional carer. This conflict, for Klein, is based in psychic fantasy and feelings of ambivalence perhaps more than in breaks in attunement between both parties.

Klein also helps us to understand some of the partly unconscious processes involved in harmful practices resonant of Kitwood's (1997) notion of malignant social psychology in dementia care. Klein clearly fleshes out the mechanisms of projection and introjection which operate

---

8 The first of these internalised objects is the part-object of the mother's breast (Klein, 1952b).

in all relationships. To return to the mother-infant pair, the mother-breast is experienced in object terms, something real while also constructed out of fantasised projections. A complex dynamic between the real external breast and the internal world of the infant takes place. The infant understands (unconsciously) the motivation of the part-object based partly on accurate perception (is the presentation of the breast responsive, withholding, anxious?). Mixed in with this is also what the infant is projecting on to it (gratitude, love, desire, rage, rejection). The infant introjects the experience of both the real breast and also her own feelings that have been projected into it. Internal objects are experienced initially as either good or bad/loved or hated, thus existing in the mind as part-objects. In part this splitting is a defensive psychic action to protect that part of the object which is loved: the loved untainted with the hated. As noted earlier, the ego, the internal world of self, is also split at this point. We might wonder how often a care worker takes on the projections of a person with dementia, left feeling that she is unable to provide satisfactory care. Or if the recipient of care takes on projections from the staff team, becoming a receptacle for disavowed feelings? How, if at all, do processes of splitting manifest themselves within the care organisation?

The 'paranoid-schizoid position' (Klein, 1946, p. 2) is characterised by a dramatic alternation between love and hate. The internal objects are both loving and hating, as is the ego. Klein's 'depressive position' (Klein, 1946, p. 14) awakens feelings of guilt. At this stage, somewhere in the child's mind, he has come to imagine that he has damaged his love objects with an over-abundance of hate. The depressive position brings about the desire to repair the relationship with both his real external objects and the internal objects within. To attain the depressive position means that the child has understood that the hated object is also the loved object. To hold such powerful feelings in check with one another signifies the child's capacity to relate to a whole human object, to show concern and to be able to integrate apparently contradictory emotional states. At the heart of this process is a more rounded, ambivalent relationship with the other (complex and paradoxical) and with the self. The Kleinian infant, having worked through the depressive position, develops a capacity for care and responsibility. The Kleinian model of development suggests that human behaviour can be brought 'back to oscillations between paranoid-schizoid and depressive positions' (Keane, 2012, p. 9). Here we see a concrete difference with Winnicott, who resisted this explanation and formulated ideas which contributed to the understanding of playful and creative states of mind, which related to the capacity for residing in paradoxical, and transitional, experience. Klein's two positions can be used to understand the dynamics both in organisations and within dyadic encounters. The paranoid-schizoid position describes mechanisms at work when feelings are split off from one source and get located in another. The depressive position, thought of as a spatial configuration, can also be a useful paradigm for reflective practice in which strong feelings can be helpfully processed and reintegrated into the care work. We might, then, talk about the depressive position involving a difficult yet helpful reparative process. Reparation, as Kosofsky Sedgwick (2007) points out, does not mean that the object is restored, as before, but that a more realistic, integrated one emerges. The depressive position comes to represent a careful handling of hate and love, and it subsequently becomes '... a uniquely spacious rubric... (a site for) Klein's explorations of intellectual creativity' (Kosofsky Sedgwick, 2007, p. 637).

Beyond this the act of reparation is often a motivating factor for doing care work, as we shall see in the course of this piece of work[9]. I would argue that this latter position is also related to the process of normal mourning, of encountering the pain of loss, and working through conflicting feelings – an experience often defended against in care work.

BION: CONTAINMENT

The works of Klein and Winnicott address the way in which the human subject develops intersubjectively through the maternal relationship, setting the scene for a model of psychic development based on the experience of security. Bion (1962b) makes a further claim about the early relationship between mother and infant. He sees this relationship as integral to the formation of the thinking mind. Bion suggests that it is within this relationship that the infant-then-child learns how to understand his own emotional experiences.

It was Bion who introduced the notion of the 'container and contained' (Bion, 1962a, p. 90). An early containing experience (offered by mother) was lacking in his psychotic patients, who relied on projective

---

9 Note the interview with care worker, Chaya, *Mothers*.

identification (in the paranoid-schizoid position) as a method of communicating their needs. Here we are reminded of Klein's influence.

Bion believed that projective identification was an interpersonal process in which the person projectively identifying 'engages in an unconscious phantasy of ejecting an unwanted aspect of him or herself... and depositing that part into another person in a controlling way' (Ogden, 1990b, p. 145). The recipient of the projective identification is driven through interpersonal pressures to behave in accordance with the split-off part of the projector now located inside herself. If the recipient (mother or analyst) is unable to contain the projection and return it in a more manageable form for re-internalisation by the projector then the recipient becomes an external threat, and the internal menace from which the projective identification sprang will remain unknown and unthought (in the projector). If the reverse happens, for the infant in the container-contained relationship, then thinking based on feeling becomes a possibility.

Bion's (1962a) model for experiential learning hinges on the mother's ability to act as a container for his projections and to make contact with the baby's state of mind. The baby has a sense of falling apart when his needs feel overwhelming. Although distressing for the mother, all being well she is nonetheless able to bear the full weight of what Bion (1962a, p. 6) calls beta-elements (pre-symbolic signals of distress). It is her alpha function (her thinking mind)[10] that processes them, returning them to the infant in a digestible form. This in turn helps the infant to begin to find ways to understand his own experience, arguably distinguishing between reality and fantasy, paving the way to separate out the conscious elements of the mind from the unconscious. The receptivity to being stirred up emotionally – what Bion would call reverie – is 'the basis of our capacity to be responsive in all occasions throughout life when we

---

10 'It seemed convenient to suppose an alpha-function to convert sense data into alpha-elements and thus provide the psyche with the material for dream thoughts, and hence the capacity to wake up or go to sleep, to be conscious or unconscious. According to this theory consciousness depends on alpha-function, and it is a logical necessity to suppose that such a function exists if we are to assume that the self is able to be conscious of itself in the sense of knowing itself from experience of itself. Yet the failure to establish, between infant and mother, a relationship in which normal projective identification is possible precludes the development of an alpha-function and therefore of a differentiation of elements into conscious and unconscious.' (Bion, 1962, p. 45)

are brought into intimate contact with someone else's state of mind' (Shuttleworth, 1989, p. 27).

In his paper, *The Psycho-analytic Study of Thinking*, Bion (1962b) suggests that the process of containment involved in mother–infant relating leads to thoughts, thinking and finally to communication of an honest or truthful nature. There is something about the notion of truthful communication that resonates, for me, with Winnicott's ideas on authenticity. Although Bion is concerned with the truthful naming of emotional experience, Winnicott is also preoccupied with the child's capacity to express emotional experience, the self, in as truthful a way as possible. Although Winnicott was not primarily focused on thinking, it is possible to recognise that both men were trying to find ways – via different avenues – to understand how some achieve an experience of authenticity[11] and others do not.

The inability to digest our emotional experiences results in a minus K (non-knowing) functioning, in which we operate defensively in order to evade what can be the pain of experience and what we might come to 'know' from it. Organisationally speaking, the space for experiential learning is often unavailable for care workers yet necessary for people to do thoughtful work (Lowe, 2014).

Paul Terry (2010) likens the care worker's role to the receptivity a parent might have in relation to the infant's needs. Terry suggests that, without the containing presence of a dementia care worker, the person with the condition can be disabled further. In other words someone must be emotionally available to the mind that ebbs away, to make sure the person concerned has an experience of being thought about while his mental processes are undergoing radical alteration.

In his seminal paper, 'Attacks on Linking', Bion (1959) argued that it was a failure in early containment experiences, and no chance of using normal projective identification, that left the infant devoid of a mind (minus-K) robust enough to process and join thoughts together in a cohesive narrative of experience. Containment helps us to reflect and learn from experience, which is important in the dementia care field because such environments can be rife with very highly charged emotional content.

---

11 In the sense of being 'me' in my own idiom, not in the image of my fantasised object.

Organisational relatedness

I do not wish to over-state my use of Menzies-Lyth's (1959) study. However, her examination of pervasive defensive practice, systematically assembled at the level of the organisational labour process, has been very influential in terms of understanding health and social care organisations at work. Her understanding has a distinctly object-relations quality to it, and though my work does not reference her study in depth, it is important to note her contribution to understanding organisational settings. Beyond this, Armstrong (2005), whose work directly informs my own, owes some of his thinking to Menzies-Lyth (1959), particularly in terms of identifying defensive organisational practice.

ARMSTRONG: ORGANISATION-IN-THE-MIND

Armstrong (2005) is interesting because his ideas span object relations, aspects of Winnicott, and also organisational consultancy traditions. His notion of the organisation-in-the-mind creatively bridges the gap between the internal world of the client and the external world – made of multiple internal worlds interacting – of the organisation at large. The notion of the organisation-in-the-mind as a psycho-social field (Armstrong, 2005 in Hoggett & Clarke, 2009, p. 246) finds echoes in Ettinger's (2006) work on the matrixial field. Here multiple traces of identity meet with the multiple traces of identity found in others, forming new identities-in-process. Her matrixial field is understood as a psychic resonance field of multiples, all interacting and generating new sets of meaning. Armstrong (2005) does not cite Ettinger in any of his work. However, what both theories demonstrate is the level of complexity involved in human relating. In a care home setting, care workers are interacting with each other, and with layers of management, as well as those in their care: giving some thought to the way that they might conceptualise the organisation-in-the-mind affords them the opportunity to test the reality of each individual conception, and also to see their contribution to it.

As Armstrong (2005a) points out, 'emotional experience is very rarely located within a purely individual space' (p. 32). If we relate this to organisational life, we come to understand that the organisation is bound up with the individual identities within it. How each one of us understands organisational life, its structures, routines and practices, is personal, tied up with our own emotional lives. In all organisations, this is taking place, but in care organisations where the work itself stirs up a great deal of powerful emotion, it is undoubtedly important to offer care workers the space to tease out what belongs to them as individuals and what might belong to the system as a whole.

The work of clinical psychoanalysis is the exploration of the phenomena that take place dynamically between the pair; in group work the object of study becomes the phenomena that take place between more than two people, also relating to both internal and external realities in dynamic interaction. By paying close attention to these phenomena, it is possible to begin to see the way that the group-in-the-mind or 'organisation-in-the-mind' (Armstrong, 2005a) is constructed between and within a membership. The emotional reality of the organisation as a whole is then registered within the individual in role. As Hutton et al (1997) write:

> 'Organisation-in-the-mind' is what the individual perceives in his or her head of how activities and relations are organised, structured and connected internally. It is a model internal to oneself, part of one's inner world, relying upon the inner experiences of my interactions, relations and the activities I engage in, which give rise to images, emotions, values and responses in me, which may consequently be influencing my own management and leadership, positively or adversely.
>
> (Quoted in Armstrong, 2005a, p. 4)

What Armstrong's work makes clear is that in order to improve organisational life, to allow teams to function with greater openness to experience, people need a 'third space' (Benjamin, 2007; 2018; Britton, 1989; Diamond, 2007; Lowe, 2014), or a potential space (Winnicott, 1971; Ogden, 1990), in which to think about the 'organisation-in-the-mind' of the team and of the individual. The process of constructing this third space often involves the complex coming together of different, sometimes tense, constellations of emotional experiences. It is also coloured by the various mechanisms, such as projective identification, introjection and splitting, that people use to deal with those experiences.

For Armstrong (2005b),

> To work analytically in groups, or in institutions, is to use one's alertness to the emotional experience presented in such settings as the medium

for seeking to understand, formulate and interpret the relatedness *of the individual to the group or the institution. It is understanding that relatedness, I believe, which liberates the energy to discover what working and being in the group or the institution can become.*

(p. 1)

Of the individuals he consults with, he treats each one as a person-in-role within the system. Armstrong seeks to understand this position as an expression of the individual's relatedness to the organisation, as an expression of the organisation in his mind. This position is 'a facet of the emotional experience that is contained within the inner psychic space of the organisation and the interactions of its members — the space between' (2005b, p. 1). The organisation-in-the-mind is an object of exploration that, at times, might facilitate one's understanding about malignant forms of social psychology, as conceptualised by Kitwood.

BRITTON: TRIANGULAR SPACE

The notion of a space inside and between minds is highly valued in psychoanalytical literature. Space allows the analyst and the analysand, mother and baby, the opportunity to do thinking work based on feeling work.

I will briefly consider Britton's (1989) work on the relationship of the child to the parental coupling as a useful frame to think about the roles that people take up in organisations. Britton's ideas draw from the Freudian concept of the Oedipal complex, and although others from different schools of thought write extensively about third/triangular/ potential spaces (Benjamin, 2007; 2018; Diamond, 2007; Winnicott, 1971; Ogden, 1990; Lowe, 2014) Britton's theory is clearly embedded within the 'organisational' frame of the family, moving out from the dyadic encounter. His theory of thirds, as well as other conceptual approaches to spatially conceived thinking processes, is linked to my belief that the third space is one that ought to be formally written in to organisational practice.

To return to Britton, he points out that a child needs to become aware of his role within the family constellation, and recognise that the parental coupling is distinct from parental-child coupling. The former is procreative and genital; the latter is not. The internalisation of the primal scene as a creative gift, rather than as an attacking presence, has, in Britton's view, implications for the way we make connections and links as we move through the life course. The coming-together of the parents in the mind brings unity to a child's psychic world. A link is formed which joins the parents, and two separate links connecting the child to each parent, creating a 'triangular space' (Britton, 1989; 1998; 2004).

Those links provide a mental space within the boundary of a triangle where separate relationships between different configurations of objects exist. Although in the primary family triangle the parental link is at first experienced as excluding the child, if he is able to tolerate the link and become curious about it, he will find himself in a third position in which he becomes a witness to a relationship beyond him while also being witnessed himself from different vantage points and in different relationships. In this sense, the infant is making links and associations in his mind. Linking is also a feature of Bion's (1962) work, as this for him is the bedrock of a thinking mind. There is also possibly some connection with Winnicott's (1971) idea of the potential space here, in which associations can be made freely and spontaneously, where the infant can also experience the paradoxical components of himself. In Britton's model, the child, viewing himself from different angles, might begin to see himself as made up of continuous and discontinuous aspects of identity, although this is not stated explicitly. Here we might see its relevance to caring organisations, where, given the closeness and proximity of the care worker to the person with dementia, it might sometimes be hard to find on a daily basis a third dimension which allows staff to view themselves outside of the immediacy of the task. Finally, Benjamin (2018), whose conception of the Third is about the practice of relating rather than thinking, states:

> *Thinking of the Third as a position draws from and bears resemblance to Klein's formulation of the depressive position, in which we can accept within ourselves a host of binaries including that of doer and done to. But in my usage it is meant to describe the state of the relationship, the stance towards real others, not to representations of internal objects... As form, the third position designates both a kind of relationship and its organising principle... The function of such a relationship... is to serve as the basis for lawful relationship to other humans, to enable recognition of the other, to move us out of tendencies to control and submission.*
>
> (p. 78)

I wish to emphasise this quote because among analysts who make use of the notion of the third or a potential space, there are those who use it to make sense of the internal object landscape, and one's role in it (Britton), and those who use such notions to describe a function of healthy and creative human relating *to real persons* (Benjamin; Winnicott). I have at times referred to both ways of conceptualising thirds. From an organisational perspective, in terms of understanding oneself in role, Britton's third proves most useful.

Applying his idea to the organisation, what we might be talking about is the capacity to stand outside of oneself to think about one's role in relation to others. *How am I seen and what can I see in myself?* Such a position also offers a unique perspective for learning about oneself in the world or in the organisation. *What are my particular emotional contributions to the organisational dynamic? What does the organisation put into me?* The third space is a concept that has particular relevance for organisations, enabling professionals to make links between their own behaviours and their work, individually and collectively. If workers are able to think about themselves in these terms, there may be the potential for avoiding splitting off disavowed feelings and projecting them into others, a process which may lead to relationships which involve the power-play of subjugation and dominance.

Holding Time is indebted to different strands of psychoanalytic theory and adopts a theoretically pluralistic approach. From Winnicott, I take, in particular, the notions of holding and the potential space that emerges in play; from Klein, the processes of splitting and rupture and repair; from Ettinger, the idea of a trans-subjective form of relating that precedes the verbal and which has paradoxically provided me with a linguistic frame to understand such moments; from Bion, his careful understanding of the need for containing raw emotion both at an individual and systemic level; from Armstrong the organisation-in-the-mind; and from Britton a conceptualisation of space which involves observing oneself in relation to others, learning about role and responsibility in the organisation.

Applying theory in this way has meant that my thinking on Winston Grove and Whittinghall is unlikely to provide the reader with a conclusive and complete statement on what was happening in the care home sites of Winston Grove and Whittinghall. Rather, I hope that by employing this approach there will be room for further thought – gaps which offer up a potential space not only for further thinking but also one which may allow those of us in the caring professions to recognise the inconsistencies and difficult paradoxes we may encounter in the work, as well as gaining some understanding of some of the causes of the malignant social psychology that Kitwood noted in dementia care.

As Winnicott states:

> *My contribution is to ask for a* paradox *to be accepted and tolerated and respected, and for it not to be resolved. By* flight *to split-off intellectual functioning it is possible to resolve the* paradox, *but the price of this is the loss of the value of* paradox *itself.*
>
> (Winnicott, 1971, xii).

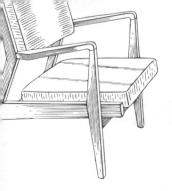

WINSTON GROVE

A chill is in the air and leaves, rusty-coloured and crisp, have long-since fallen to the pavements; a child dressed in thick layers is whizzing down a slide in the playpark opposite while his mother looks on. People are shopping and stopping at cafes on the high street a few minutes' walk from Winston Grove. Inside the forty-bedded home for older people, we know that Autumn is here, too, from the bright orange notice on the door to the activities room, 'Happy Halloween'. Another wall is decorated with Halloween faces and in the background, despite the room being empty, there is music from the sixties playing.

But this is not where Daphne is. She is walking past the main reception area of the home, where two bright red and white striped sofas in a corduroy fabric are positioned adjacent to one another. Sometimes residents sit there and chat, or simply watch who is coming and going through the main door. Occasionally they notice the fish tank that is placed in front of the window, right next to the sofas. Today there are no residents seated, though there is evidence of people living lives and leaving mess, symbolised in the pair of trousers draped on top of the fish tank, partly obscuring the fish. On top of one of the sofa's cushions is a packet of digestives, with several biscuits escaping.

We might think Daphne is trying to escape, to get outside and take a walk on the common past the badminton courts that offer one approach to Winston Grove. Or she might want to turn left and walk towards the high street, stop at the local market just in front of the supermarket, head to the church on the green or even try one of the coffee shops that sells wholesome homemade bread and cakes. Daphne would probably enjoy a trip to a restaurant or the opportunity to see the children playing in the playground in the neighbouring primary school. But today Benjamin, her long-term partner, is not coming to take her out for one of her regular trips to the cinema, to a park, to lunch, and so Daphne walks past the lift on the ground floor next to the main entrance door.

Erica and the assistant manager take their leave of Daphne, and explain that they have to go into room four. A resident in that room has died. Nobody says anything further about it, but it is known. An empty room is a telling sign. People don't talk about death at Winston Grove, though people here die. Disappearances are marked by empty chairs and RIP signs scrawled on a whiteboard, but spending any time thinking about the losses of people you might actually like seems too much.

It is now up to Erica to organise the trinkets and clothes for the grieving family to pick up. With her file, and the supervision of the assistant manager, she will cross-reference what is left against the inventory noted on the residents' arrival at Winston Grove. Beyond memories, just a handful of remaining items symbolise a life that ends in the small space of room four.

'Oh ok then,' says Daphne, who lingers behind the two women. She follows them to the bedroom door but stops as they walk in. 'I am a silly sausage really. It worries me. I don't know these people well and I am being a silly sausage.' Daphne turns a little and continues walking along the corridor. 'There are some good people, nice people here and they are doing all they can to make things well. It can't be good all the time, though.' Does she know what will be discussed behind the door of room four? That the unfolding of pain is concealed there.

Daphne takes in her surroundings. She notices the photos of a female resident, one youthful, one more recent, stuck on a bedroom door, a reminder that this is her room. A reminder that everyone has a history.

'Well,' Daphne says, walking on. She moves slowly past a wall with paraphernalia from the fifties displayed. There are records, an abacus, and a large picture of Rita Hayworth. 'I've no idea why they get themselves like that,' she says of the actress. Nostalgic spaces in institutions are considered good practice in dementia care, thought to stimulate meaningful interaction and reminiscence. Daphne, befuddled by Rita's appearance, pulls a quizzical expression. She doesn't stop to ruminate but follows the corridor until she reaches a bright room, coloured in yellows and pale blues. Painted fish and birds dangle from the ceiling, a dreamscape, and here we find the Happy Halloween sign. Daphne goes in.

On a table in the centre of the room are different kinds of sweets (jelly babies, liquorice allsorts, fudge) in bowls. Like a scene from *Alice in Wonderland*, but without instruction to eat or drink, Daphne picks up four segments of chocolate orange. She tips the bowl upside down, arranging the four chocolate orange segments on top of the upside down bowl to make a diamond shape. She sees a CD on the side, and moves back to the table and puts the CD on top of the liquorice allsorts. She goes to a pile of paintings and picks up two of cats, studies them for a few minutes. 'Here they are,' she says, as if she has found something she has been looking for. She places them in the middle of the table with the sweets, surveys the room as if to check that everything is now in its rightful place, in order, and leaves.

She walks out of the door, stops still, noticing that there is an open door leading to another lounge she hadn't seen before. Through the opening of the door, three residents are seen sleeping, deeply, in their chairs. Daphne whispers, 'It is a new world but an old world.' A phrase so apt. She turns her head and carries on walking, deep in thought. 'What is this life, if full of care, we have no time to stop and stare?' Daphne brings forth from the recesses of her mind these words of WH Davies. This is one of these things, she says, that come back to her. She looks through the windows to a patioed area where a metre-high fountain with two lovers under a tree takes central place. Sentimental as it is, Daphne only notices the rain.

She turns right and stops. She assesses another image of one of the residents, stuck on coloured yellow card, Blu-tacked to the front of a bedroom door. There is a photo of a family together, smiling, the resident in the middle of the picture. 'There together,' says Daphne.

Soon Daphne returns to her usual room and takes a seat again by a table in the dining room. Later loud pop music, coming from an unknown source, interrupts Daphne's reflective state. Underneath the table, she is kicking against one of its legs. She has wound her fingers together, making a giant fist out of both of her hands.

'I don't like this. Boom, boom, boom, bum, bum, bum,' says Daphne, talking about the jarring music. She teases her hands apart and puts her forefinger partially into her mouth, biting lightly down on her finger as if this is an act of self-regulation. Her eyes are still soft as she follows the resident she recognises as Mum. 'She is so kind. Always trying to help people.' You might think Daphne is talking about herself, too.

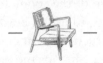

The lively high street with its tapas bars, Thai and Vietnamese cafes, high-end restaurants, boutique clothes shops, traditional boozers, seems a world away from the quieter residential road where we find Winston Grove. But that is London, different terrains, a patchwork of experiences, colours, sounds, bound together, some ill-fitting, and some seamlessly flowing into one another. Entering Winston Grove, you might imagine the contrast between the buzzing high street and the home to be a stark one; you might imagine a resident slumped in the corridor sleeping by the fish tank, today uncovered, no trousers upon it.

It's true that the place isn't immediately welcoming. To get in, there is an outside buzzer which when pressed is heard in the office. A petite woman, Wend, dressed tidily in a white blouse and black trousers, with hair cropped to her head, then presses the entry buzzer from her office. The outer door can be pushed open, giving access to the inner door that leads directly into the reception. Visitors find themselves wedged between two doors, the inner and the outer, nudging the inner door open with one foot while they fill in the visitors' log book. There were no visitors listed today, just a list of the staff – both permanent and temporary – on the morning shift.

Erica had not signed in today. The week before, despite her playfulness with Daphne, she had been clutching her back as she walked. Erica had been in pain; the work, as the activities co-ordinator once said, was literally back-breaking. Without Erica, there was no named keyworker as a point of contact to track down Daphne. Daphne would be given over to the unit, the responsibility of keyworking shared. Whether Daphne noticed a change like this was unclear, but it did suggest that structurally Daphne was even more at sea. Erica was, from this day on, signed off work and would not return. Sickness, absence, and staff turnover were issues for Winston Grove, as they were for many care organisations. The cost of working day in, day out in a physically and emotionally demanding job, with very little reward, at least financially, took its toll on many workers. With overarching cuts carers felt more undervalued. In the local borough, they'd seen nearly a million pound reduction to the recent budget, and though the spend for older people was often proportionally higher than for other vulnerable groups, Erica and her colleagues felt this was not good enough. Erica was in great physical pain but you might also wonder whether the general lack of concern for her, and the work, also had a paralysing effect.

Finding Daphne was sometimes like a treasure hunt. Given her physical mobility and accompanying desire to move freely about the home, it could be hard to find her. Daphne liked to find activity, people, which would take her to all the public spaces in the home. The only areas she couldn't access were the kitchens and staff room, found along a key-coded corridor, the only areas free from interruption. The other inaccessible area was the laundry rooms where Bridget, one of the housekeepers and breakfast assistants, found herself after she had completed the breakfast rush.

Daphne is at the edge of a large group of seated residents – almost fifteen people, made up of men and women. Dressed in a polka-dot skirt with a blouse and green cardigan, she watches the group. She is a peripheral figure. One man sits with his back towards the television, which isn't on. A line of residents in red velvety armchairs sit, backs towards the window which looks out onto part of the garden where the shed that houses the incontinence pads stands. Two rows of residents are in the middle of the room, between two sets of columns appearing to hold the ceiling up, sitting opposite each other. 'Bring me sunshine in your smile…' booms out from the CD player in the corner. Although the music brings a smile to the faces of some, others are sleeping through, inactive.

Daphne is dancing, the only resident moving backwards and forwards. She has a bright red plastic tambourine in her hand, shaking it up and down as she moves from her right foot to her left.

The activities co-ordinator, Gemma, is in the middle of the two rows of residents, putting three hoopla targets in a straight line. She bends down and moves in close towards one of the residents, asking her to stand up. The woman joins in, throwing large red, yellow, and blue plastic hoops. Daphne is shaking her tambourine vigorously, in the centre of the room. She is smiling and singing the occasional word, '… should be more happiness'. Daphne seeks out Gemma, who is trying to help balance the woman throwing the hoops by pressing her hand into the small of her back gently. Daphne stands close by, clapping her hands together when the lady throws a hoop over the stick, 'Well done,' she shouts, encouragingly. 'Lovely dancing, Daphne,' Gemma. 'Is it?' she asks.

Changing direction, Daphne walks to the other side of the room, shaking her tambourine in front of some of the residents as if to entertain them. One of the women sitting down tries to reach for the tambourine.

A male carer goes to take the tambourine from Daphne, who gives it to him unquestioningly. He then passes it to the woman who begins to use it. Sharing takes on a fluidity, thanks to Daphne's lack of resistance.

Daphne walks back to the main action. Another resident is standing up, throwing the hoops. One falls by Daphne's foot, which she picks up and holds above her head. 'I do like your halo, Daphne,' says Gemma, smiling. 'Oh, thank you,' says Daphne, laughing. Daphne reaches for the halo and pulls it down further over her head to make a necklace. Gemma approaches Daphne, asking if she can have the hoop for the resident who is playing. 'Oh I see,' says Daphne, handing it to Gemma, who finds another tambourine and gives that one to Daphne. The way Gemma swaps one object for another is instinctive. Unlike the red plastic tambourine, this one is made of wood, dried skin pulled taut around it. Daphne puts that one on her head too, giggling from time to time.

To the side of Daphne, a male carer who has been watching the scene unfold for some time looks bemused, shakes his head.

'Fly me to the moon...' the music plays on. Daphne walks toward the hoopla game, almost knocking a target down. She bends down and starts to pull the stick from its base. 'Excuse me, Daphne,' says Gemma. 'Ooh, sorry, love. I am a silly sausage,' she says. Daphne raises the stick in the air with one hand, holding the tambourine with the other. She twirls it around and around, enjoying herself, forgetting that a moment ago she was concerned about being a silly sausage.

Gemma explains to Daphne that she needs the stick for the game. Daphne looks her in the eyes, smiling, and hands it back. Gemma gives Daphne a hug, placing her arm around Daphne's shoulders. 'Thank you very much.'

Gemma moves around the circle of residents, offering each resident a turn on the hoopla. Daphne walks towards a sideboard where there are a variety of objects. She stops at a cardboard display of 3D trees and picks them up. She pops them on her head. She walks through a small space between two men, still holding the trees on her head, making her way back to the hoopla game.

'Are you having a good time?' asks Gemma. 'I am. This is what it is,' she says.

Gemma signals the end of the activity by turning the music down. Understanding that the party is over, Daphne goes to find a seat and sits down very slowly. She is quiet, watching Gemma speak with some other residents who have come downstairs. She asks them if they want to go back upstairs. All of them do. Three residents get up one by one with Gemma's support and follow her slowly, with their frames.

Minutes pass until Gemma returns to the room and asks the remaining residents if anyone would like to see the guinea pigs upstairs. Daphne agrees. Two other residents get up. Daphne follows, very quiet now. No one speaks. Tiredness is in the air. In the lift, one resident mentions that it is a squash.

The lift doors open at the second floor. Gemma leads the residents into a lounge and asks them to wait a moment. Daphne sits herself down slowly, holding the armrests tightly as she lowers herself, yawning. Gemma comes back into the room with a guinea pig, cradled in her arms. She puts it in front of Daphne. 'I know, little one,' Daphne says. 'It is like this. You are a good one, and it will be all right. I am sure one day it will be good for you. What a lovely one. I think that is all I can say today.'

Meanwhile another carer has been looking for Daphne. 'There you are, Daphne. Oh but you need to be downstairs. Benjamin is coming any minute.' 'Oh, I see,' says Daphne, worn out, unenthusiastic.

'You will need a coat,' says the carer. She helps Daphne, puzzled, out of the chair. As they walk towards her bedroom to get a coat, Daphne is confused. 'They bring me here, there. I go one way. It's all meaningless, I'm sure.'

The carer opens Daphne's bedroom door and goes in. She holds it ajar with Daphne outside. 'Come on then, Daphne,' the carer says, coat in her arm. 'Let's wait for Benjamin and the taxi.'

'But I am tired now,' says Daphne.

'You will be fine. I'm sure you will enjoy it, Daphne. It is a beautiful day. You will have lunch out, maybe go to the pictures.'

They get to the lift; the carer presses the button. Daphne walks to the back of the lift and sits herself down. The lift door opens. The carer shows Daphne a seat in reception where the fish tank is and asks her to sit there for a few minutes until Benjamin comes. Daphne strikes up a brief conversation with two ladies who have been in reception all morning. 'I can sit here?' asks Daphne, politely. 'Of course you can,' they say.

Daphne waits patiently, holding her coat in her lap. The doorbell buzzes and a tall man and a lady come in. They explain that they are helping Benjamin, who we know is very frail himself. This is why Daphne is living at Winston Grove. Benjamin's physical condition meant that he could not give her the care she needed as her dementia progressed. Nonetheless, as regular as clockwork, he makes his weekly visit to take his partner out, to places they once enjoyed together.

From Winston Grove Daphne will pass the high street and continue a few miles further, closing in on the banks of the river, eventually stopping at a friendly arts centre, which houses a cafe, gallery, theatre, and cinema. This was once part of Daphne's thriving world and Benjamin hopes she will still take pleasure in it with him, possibly as much as she had enjoyed her earlier dance.

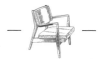

Some days were quiet. Without distractions at Winston Grove, Daphne was left to be with herself. On these occasions it was harder for her to summon up the energy to engage with staff members and other residents. It can be difficult to be alone; for some people sleep was the only response; for others walking away physically from the discomfort helped. It was on a day like this, when residents were either withdrawing through sleep or wandering the corridors, restless, that, unannounced, an inspector had visited. Gemma was out of the building, a day off. No alternative activities had been timetabled, so there was no way of masking those moments of painful solitude. The manager, Elaine, was at meetings all day. She was a lively manager, someone who got her hands dirty when the home needed her.

Senior management was low on the ground, the number of senior care workers at half the required number. A few weeks before a new face, a senior, had begun work only to have left a week later, claiming that her commute was too far. So the day the inspector came there was a skeleton staff team and, without Gemma, an absence of structured activity.

The inspector had spent the full day at Winston Grove. She'd noted the usual shortcomings: a broken cupboard, still unseen to, and a couple of care plans in need of update. But what had concerned her most were two care workers – one permanent, the other temporary – who had spoken brusquely to two residents. They hadn't offered enough choice; hadn't used residents' first names either.

Winston Grove was not looking good: under-staffed and inactive. The inspection had made Elaine and Wend anxious. Service Managers knew about the shortcomings but, until then, no one had acted. Winston Grove had been left to its own devices, which suited the home in some ways; undermined it in others. Elaine joked from time to time that she was glad that the inspector hadn't found all of the animals: the dog, the visiting stray cat, the birds, and the guinea pigs. Now she might be able to bring a horse in too! But she was concerned about the future of Winston Grove. Cuts were all around her, and one home was likely to be closed in the borough, following the closure of a local day centre, and a library. Despite the demographic profile and anticipated mental health needs in the borough being predicted to rise, closures were still forecast. She doubted it would be Winston Grove because of its location, though one unit was not full. This was because of the push to keep people with dementia in the community until the bitter end. The headline numbers for the borough showed that fewer older people in the borough were moved into residential care whereas many more, over 2,000, were supported to stay at home. Of course, there would always be the fear that any inspection downgrading could be terminal. The home had, after all, been well rated in the past.

Today was one of those days when Winston Grove did not look like the best place for Daphne, who was listless and disengaged, relying on her own resources. Daphne is sitting in a seat, her back facing a courtyard. Behind her a chicken has mounted a wall. She is next to an older woman, Suki, who often calls out for help to go to the toilet. This woman has a food bib around her neck, a stack of biscuits on a table next to her, her feet up on a stool in front of her.

Daphne is looking straight ahead towards the television. There is a programme on – someone is hunting down antiques. Daphne is sitting still in her chair, frowning momentarily from behind her glasses. Daphne wears a black blouse with small white flowers on it, a green cardigan and navy pleated skirt. Her feet are crossed, but she is tapping the bottom foot on the ground.

She turns to the lady sitting next to her then returns her gaze to the television, letting out a silent sigh. Her arms are wrapped around her waist, crossed. Her chin juts out almost imperceptibly. It's as if Daphne is holding herself together, arms around body, quite still. She stretches out both legs, straightens them, tapping the right foot on the floor.

Bridget, in a dark brown cleaning top, comes in, smiling at Daphne. 'Hey ho,' says Daphne weakly. 'Hey ho,' Bridget says back with little energy, walking into the kitchen. Daphne follows the cleaner with her eyes for a moment before looking back at the television.

'Benjamin is not saying a lot today,' says Daphne. She is referring to the old woman next to her, mistaking her for her long-term partner. No one is saying a lot today. 'It's been a nice quiet morning,' says Daphne. With that she begins to stand.

Daphne makes her way out of the lounge, turning left to the main reception. She walks past the office where the manager and senior duty staff are discussing a way to increase the training for staff. Gemma walks past with another resident, guiding her with a frame. 'Hey ho,' says Daphne. 'Hey ho,' says Gemma. Fleeting moments of connection are followed by disconnection, and Daphne is walking, walking, walking.

A woman with red socks walks behind Daphne and appears to be struggling to use the lift. She realises that there is a door to upstairs and goes up. A woman sitting in reception is making bemused expressions as she watches the resident in the red socks. Daphne looks at the fish in the fish tank. 'Nothing changes really, though it is still interesting. It is,' she says forlornly. 'There are not enough children here, though.'

A resident is having her hands massaged by one of the carers. She says that it's nice that they are helping one another.

'The parents don't want to hear it sometimes. At least, no arguments,' she says. Daphne gets up, the idea of conflict perhaps unsettling her? A carer is writing care plans. Daphne stops there for some time. 'How are you, Daphne?' the carer asks. Daphne would like to be of help, although she is worried about being silly. She wants to be of use but fears she will fail. 'You have nothing to be worried about; you are entitled to be yourself, Daphne,' says the carer. She asks Daphne to find peace in herself. A remark kind and thoughtless at the same time.

Daphne turns to me, still worried about appearing daft. I can see how concerned she is. She turns to me and raises her eyebrows, ever so softly. 'You are helping me,' she says, and I wonder what I am doing.

The older woman, Suki, whom Daphne was originally sitting next to is covered in a blanket. She also wants help. She demands it. 'Oi, you must help me.' A carer walks into the room and stops, then bows forward with both hands pressed together. 'How can I help you, Suki?' she says. 'I want cake,' she says.

'Ok, let me check.' She goes to the back of the room and asks the carer in charge, who is folding napkins for lunch. 'No, if she has more cake now, she will not eat any lunch.' Here you might be reminded of mothers and children. The carer explains that pudding will be coming after lunch.

'I hope you aren't going to fall asleep here now and start snoring. It puts me off,' says the carer in charge, harshly. She is speaking to a woman who is already at the dining table, looking sleepy.

'I want more cake,' shouts Suki. A temporary carer who is helping an old man to sit back down in his chair, placing a bib around his neck, turns, and shouts back. 'It's your lunch soon.' As she walks away her voice becomes less audible. 'I'll be there on the double.'

'This sort of thing is so very rude.' Daphne is unimpressed by the shouting. 'I blame the people that employ the people,' she says. 'What sort of politeness is this? I don't like it at all.' It was in this unit that the inspector had noticed the abrupt manner of the care staff.

The carer goes back to Suki, places her lunch in front of her on a small table with wheels. Suki's assertiveness means that she gets what she wants, often before quieter others. Eventually, after ten minutes' waiting, a carer retrieves Daphne from her seat. 'Come and sit down with the ladies,' she says to Daphne. The carer pulls out a chair and invites Daphne to sit down. Daphne walks to the other side of the table, pulling out another chair in between two other residents.

'Oh, can't we get out of here?' says Daphne, introducing herself to the table.

The carer places lunch in front of Daphne, who begins eating while staring towards the kitchen. She is not looking at her food. Instead she focuses on a scene in which Bridget is attending to a woman, slouched in her chair, and feeding her patiently. Food as a symbol of care, pleasure, sustenance could be mistreated at Winston Grove. Sometimes it was withheld, and used in a play for power. Other times it was presented beautifully on the plate. Sometimes residents took it into their bodies happily; other times the nourishment was rejected. Lunchtimes could become sites of calm or tension, just like mealtimes in families where competing needs played out around the table.

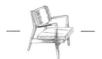

Friendships were forged, also forgotten. Sometimes friendships seemed to be based on temporal misalignments or misrecognised identities. Sometimes it was important to be close to someone, wandering corridors looking for home; sometimes friendships like these quickly turned hostile. Friendships were rarely sustained. Winston Grove – despite all its attempts to build community – didn't have the time to support them.

Daphne is walking in the corridor with another tall, slender resident by her side. Daphne is in one of her pleated skirts; the other resident in black trousers, her short hair a little dishevelled. The tall woman presses her hand gently into the small of Daphne's back. They are walking in the direction of the activities room, following a number of other residents guided by a young volunteer with a headscarf on. Daphne and her friend walk past a toilet, the door slightly ajar. 'That is the one… that's open,' says Daphne. The friend mumbles.

They continue walking past the toilet, turning the corner, past the 1950s wall. No comment. They walk past another toilet to the right. This door is opened further. A man is putting the toilet seat down. Another resident is walking towards them, stooped, her head looking down at the floor and both of her hands jiggling out in front of her. Everyone stops. The friend says something inaudible. The other resident moves her head upwards, making eye contact.

'Oh yes, well here she is,' Daphne says to her friend.

'She is,' says the friend.

'Best not to get too involved,' says Daphne, possibly sensing a difference in posture between her and the woman she has just passed. The two friends walk into an activities room where the volunteer has set up space for a number of residents to paint images of Christmas presents.

'Do you want to sit here?' asks the volunteer, ushering Daphne into a seat. 'Do you want me to?' asks Daphne, unsure. 'Yes, you could do if you'd like to.' Daphne sits down but keeps herself back in her chair, away from the materials in front of her.

'What is this?' asks Daphne. The volunteer explains that she can paint the image in front of her if she wishes to. Daphne's friend is looking perplexed, angry, standing behind Daphne to the left. The friend picks up the paper and shuffles it around in front of Daphne. 'This is for kids,' she says, furiously.

'You don't want to do it?' Daphne asks her friend. 'It's for kids,' she repeats. She picks up a small bowl full of glittery shapes and walks towards a large window with them. She empties them on the floor.

She stands behind Daphne again, and bends down towards her and presses her hand on the left hand side of Daphne's chest. She begins to pull slightly on Daphne's black cardigan. 'Come on,' she says.

Daphne crunches up her eyebrows, forming a frown. 'What shall I do?' Daphne asks the volunteer. The volunteer invites her to paint, demonstrating what the other residents are doing. The volunteer is by herself in the room, without any permanent members of staff. She is young, a college student, studying health and social care at a sixth form college close by. She is patient but seems ill-equipped to deal with the tension that is mounting in the room.

The friend pulls at Daphne's cardigan. 'Come on', more forcefully this time. 'Get off me,' says Daphne. 'Just leave me be.' The friend puts her hands over one of the photocopied images of presents. 'For kids,' she says angrily. She walks towards the door and stops, then walks back towards Daphne.

Daphne looks anxious. She is not painting but the volunteer gently tries to encourage her. 'For kids,' shouts the other lady. 'Oh please,' says Daphne, 'don't speak at the same time. I have one rude person shouting and another politely asking what I think.' Daphne looks at a loss. She stands up and begins to leave the room. 'Thank you,' she says to the volunteer gratefully, but loyal to her increasingly frustrated friend.

They walk back the way they came, stopping momentarily. Daphne's friend sees some books left on a huge bookcase and flicks through one of them. Daphne lets go, as if dropping her friend off, walking past the fish tank in reception and into the lounge where she usually has breakfast, lunch, and dinner. She walks to the back of the room to the double doors which open onto the gardens. She pats down the curtains. She opens them slightly then closes them tight again. She takes the material in her hand and studies it. 'What's she fiddling about with there?' asks one of the residents sitting in the lounge. No one answers.

A carer walks towards Daphne, asking her if she is all right. 'I'd do anything for a drink,' she says. 'What would you like, Daphne? A cup of tea?' Daphne agrees and follows the carer into the kitchen. The carer notices that all the teacups are in the dishwasher so nips next door to borrow one. 'There they are,' says Daphne, noticing the chickens outside. She watches them for a moment and then leaves the kitchen, back into the corridor again. She walks past several bedrooms, holding her hands in front together, anxiously. She walks full circle and appears back in the lounge. She notices a blanket on one of the chairs and begins to unfold it. She studies the pattern, folds it in half and in half again.

The carer who had gone to find a cup has made Daphne a cup of tea. 'Daphne, I have a tea for you.'

'Oh lovely,' says Daphne. She looks lost. 'Benjamin is fast asleep,' says Daphne, as if she needs to find someone to anchor her.

Daphne sits down, staring ahead. She picks up her tea, holding it there for a while. The carer asks her if she would like sugar. 'Yes, please,' says Daphne, face softening.

The carer goes to get a bowl of sugar and places it in front of Daphne, 'Here you are, Daphne.'

Daphne takes the spoon from the sugar bowl and scoops up a teaspoon of sugar. She stirs the sugar in and begins drinking her tea. Silently, she puts her tea down and scoops up another teaspoon of sugar. This time she puts the sugar straight into her mouth and eats it.

All of a sudden there is loud shouting in the corridor. One resident's voice is louder than another. 'She's cross, that one,' says one of the residents. Daphne's friend has just thrown a ball at the head of another resident. The senior carer appears and stands in the middle of them. 'You mustn't throw things at people.' Daphne is watching. She has a puzzled expression as if she is trying to work out where she knows the woman from. The deputy manager can be heard asking the other resident not to inflame the situation. She asks them to part ways as they don't get on well. Perhaps Daphne has had a lucky escape.

She retrieves the spoon and scoops up more sugar and eats it again.

A carer comes past and asks Daphne if she fancies having her nails done. 'Oh no,' says Daphne, 'no thanks.' She smiles sweetly at the carer. 'But what if Benjamin is coming today, Daphne, to take you out?' Romance is alive in the carer's mind. 'Oh no,' says Daphne, 'he's not coming today.'

Daphne continues to sit quiet and still, scooping up another sugar and eating it, as if the bitter taste of this morning's tensions can be alleviated this way.

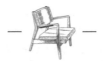

At the beginning of December, like homes all around the UK, Winston Grove was preparing for the festive season. The artificial Christmas trees were brought out of storage and one was placed in each unit, for the staff and residents to decorate. One tree was placed in reception to greet guests, acting as a permanent reminder that Christmas was upon everyone. Jim, the handyman, would hand all the decorations out in boxes to each unit. Some trees were dressed in blues and whites, others reds and greens, another golden. The decorations were vibrant and no tree was scantily clad. December was the month of the home's Christmas party and this year would be no different. Relatives would be invited; sherry, wine, mince pies, and a spread from the kitchen would be available. Dancing and a pantomime act from a touring theatrical company would follow.

Whether Benjamin had come to take Daphne to the shops to do a spot of shopping or not, he has just returned her in time for lunch. A carer opens the door to Daphne and welcomes her in. Daphne, puzzled, turns her head to the door, 'well, where is Benjamin going now?' The carer explains that he is dropping her back now and that she is welcome to have lunch. 'Oh no,' says Daphne, 'I really don't want any lunch, thank you.' The carer is not from Daphne's usual group. She is the carer of another woman, who is standing at the door with her coat on. She is waiting for her uncle, so that he will take her 'home'. The carer turns to the woman and asks her to come in the lift as lunch is ready. The woman with her coat on raises her voice, 'I am not having my lunch here, no I'm not. I thought you were my friend. No, I'm not having my lunch here.' She storms off.

Daphne is bewildered in this unfamiliar space, where people want to leave but can't or where people, like her, return but don't really want to. She turns back towards the door and asks again, 'what is Benjamin doing?' Daphne is still in a navy coat, confused following this separation, standing very still, taking in her surroundings.

The deputy manager walks up to Daphne and smiles warmly. She asks Daphne and the other woman if they are waiting to go out. 'I'm waiting for my brother now,' says the woman angrily, changing her relationship to the male she is waiting for. 'No I'm not going out,' says Daphne, perplexed. 'Oh, you have come back then, have you, Daphne? Did you have a lovely time with Benjamin?' 'Hey ho, the wind and the rain,' says Daphne sadly. 'It's nice to have you back,' says the deputy manager. She takes leave. Daphne is standing in the middle of the reception area. 'It's still here, then,' says Daphne, her gaze directed at the fish tank, a focus in the wilderness, something to hold onto. She sees the Christmas tree in the process of being dressed. She smiles gently.

'I don't know what I'm supposed to do,' says Daphne. A carer walks towards her. 'Hello, Daphne,' she says. 'Did you have a good time this morning?'

'I did, but I can't really remember what I did.'

'But you enjoyed it,' says the carer.

'Um,' Daphne says, smiling slowly, as if there is pain in the vague memory of pleasure. 'Will Benjamin come back here?'

'Benjamin knows you are here,' says the carer, 'and he comes to see you here.'

'Oh,' she says, but this doesn't seem to make sense.

The carer notices Daphne still has her coat on. 'We are about to have lunch, Daphne. Will you let me take your coat off so that you can sit and have lunch, and it'll still be kept lovely and clean, your coat, a million dollars?'

'Oh thank you, yes,' says Daphne.

The carer slowly unzips Daphne's coat and, at a careful speed and pace, takes the coat from Daphne's shoulders and brings it from her arms. The carer folds the coat and places it over her arm, and with her other arm invites Daphne to hold onto her as they walk towards the table at the back. It's as if she is keeping Daphne upright, understanding that Daphne might well be about to fall apart. 'Would you like to sit here next to the gorgeous Eunice or here opposite?' Eunice looks up briefly and looks away. Daphne makes a semi-smile and says, 'this will be all right,' and the carer pulls the chair next to Eunice and waits for Daphne to begin to manoeuvre herself down into the chair. Daphne seems to be settling, gathered up by the carer, until a workman walks in and starts talking loudly from the main kitchen, puncturing the peace that she seemed to be in need of. The carer in charge of the food trolley is getting something from a cupboard, and the workman is talking at her about his weight gain or diets in general.

All the while Daphne's head is turned in their direction, watching, her face creasing every now and again.

'Where is Diane?' asks Daphne, talking about her sister. Diane is also the name of one of the carers. The carer taking the temperatures speaks from where she is, and understands Daphne's intention. 'Diane is in an old people's home in Chester. She doesn't manage to come down to visit now as she has severe arthritis, but her daughter does come.'

'Diane is not here?' she asks. Nothing is fitting together today; people are not where she expects them to be. She is not where she expects herself to be.

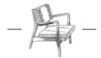

Daphne walks into the next door lounge, a room with floral lilac-coloured walls. About three residents sit in the middle of the room, on a collection of chairs positioned almost in two lines opposite one another. Towards the back of the room, three round tables have been brought close together. Gemma is speaking to five or six residents who are seated there.

At the end of one of the tables is a care worker, filling out care plans. She is seated next to a male resident. Daphne walks towards the back of the room, past a woman who looks towards her beseechingly, muttering something from her chair in a strong accent. Her body is twitching. Daphne gets closer to the residents seated by the table. Gemma gives out boards with numbers on them. She invites Daphne to sit down and play 'bingo' with everyone. Daphne sits down. A carer is fetching everyone cups of tea and coffee.

Daphne studies the board, flicking the bright red covers for each number back and forth.

Gemma picks up a wooden number from a bowl and shouts it out. She places the number in front of her on a board with all the numbers.

Daphne studies the red line of numbers, numbers up to twenty, and flicks the cover of the numbers over them from time to time. Next to Daphne, on the left, is a woman in a wheelchair, shaking. She is seated next to a carer who is helping her. This carer, who had been doing the care plans, is also helping the man seated to her left, who is concentrating.

'Legs eleven,' calls out Gemma. Daphne stares at her board but doesn't do anything. 'Never quite sure, number four, I'll try to rhyme them,' says Gemma. Daphne laughs. She has the number four and her finger hovers over it for a few seconds. Gemma notices Daphne considering whether or not she is right, and says, 'That's the one, Daphne.' Daphne pulls the cover over the number. She reaches for her cup of coffee and takes a sip of the drink. She slowly puts it back down as Gemma takes out another number, 'Happy to be alive, number fifty-five.' Daphne smiles again, a bigger grin this time. She looks to the woman next to her, who is worried about whether she has fifty-five or not. Gemma bends down and helps, explaining that she is right.

'Where's the milk?' asks a male resident. The carer explains that the milk is in the jug in front of him. He smiles up at her, making eye contact, thanks her, and begins pouring his milk.

Daphne pushes her chair under the table and begins to walk out of the lounge. She notices a Christmas tree in the corner of the room, decorated with red baubles and green baubles, and silver tinsel. 'Fascinating this is, isn't it, but I don't much like it,' she says. She leaves the room and goes back into the corridor, taking a turn left into her usual lounge with its velvety chairs, blue and gold wallpaper. She spots the Christmas tree in this room to the side of the television. This tree has been redecorated by a resident, apparently in a fit of rage, with tinsel strewn over the tree haphazardly. A maverick festive moment.

'This is a lovely place for the children,' Daphne says, looking at the tree. She turns to the window and looks at some of the courtyard decorations outside. 'It is so nice that they can have all this. This must be someone's home,' she says, recognising that it isn't hers. There is an image of an open fire on a laptop. 'What a lively place this is,' says Daphne, noticing the image. 'It really is good for them, the children.' She hears one of the carers call out to the carer, Diane. 'And Diane is here, too,' she says, comforted.

Daphne spots a toy baby doll. She sits down in the armchair next to the doll, dressed in a spotty pink dress and bright pink cardigan. She gently picks it up from its seat and puts the doll on her lap. 'He is a sweet soul,' says Daphne. 'Someone's put something there,' she says, pointing at a button on the doll's cardigan. She takes the doll in her hands, looking into its eyes. 'Aren't you a special little one? Isn't he?' She looks quite the mother now.

Daphne puts the doll back gently in a new position, with its back resting on the back of the chair now. 'You can see the room better now,' she says, knowing it's important to see things.

Daphne sits down next to a woman who seems to be deep in thought. It is nearly lunchtime. Daphne starts talking about her sister Diane being here and there. She talks about how her sister looked after her own children so well. 'Just like they always do,' someone says. The carer who had been pushing the trolley offers Daphne a plate of fish, chips, and peas. Daphne picks up one chip and dips it in a cup of blackcurrant juice. Diane sits down next to a woman who has a glazed look on her face. She may have had a stroke. Very slowly Diane cuts the woman's fish and slowly brings it to her mouth. The woman opens her mouth and takes in the piece of fish, chewing slowly. 'I'm glad you're eating,' says Diane.

Daphne watches the woman being fed and a faraway smile comes over her face. 'This is really quite a good place,' she says, as if she has seen some good enough mothering already today.

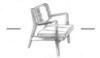

The following week, Daphne was struggling with a bad cold and felt very fragile. In this instance, summoning up the carapace of wellness, of robustness, of independence was impossible. She wanted to be mothered, as we all do when our bodies and minds no longer offer much structure to our lives. At times like these, Daphne could not be distracted from her discomfort. Gemma's lively programme of activities were not appropriate. A quiet, warm space with an attentive person was all she seemed to need.

Daphne is seated at the head of three tables, all pushed closely together. There are six residents in the room seated around the tables. Music is playing in the background. One resident is tapping her hands to the slow beat of the music. Daphne is looking down at a pink paper dragonfly, with shapes on the upper and lower wings. A man is seated next to Daphne with a yellow striped butterfly in front of him. Daphne is wearing a grey and white striped linen blouse, with a grey wrap-around cardigan and some new glasses. All of a sudden her upper body shivers.

Gemma walks into the room with her hand pressed gently into the back of one of the residents, the woman who had had a stroke before

Christmas. She is walking well and chatting. She smiles at Daphne just before she bends her legs and moves into the chair.

Gemma brings out paint palettes from a cupboard and places them between Daphne and the woman to her right, then six paints, and begins to squeeze each one onto each palette dish. She brings out a cup set of paintbrushes. One woman confidently picks up a paintbrush and begins painting an insect.

The man next to Daphne asks what he is to do. Gemma explains. He takes up the brush and begins painting. Daphne shudders. 'I have no idea about this, don't know what I am supposed to do.'

The woman who had the stroke picks up her paintbrush and begins to paint the tips of the fingers on her right hand.

One woman has fallen asleep. Another opposite Daphne begins to close her eyes. One resident is listening to the music, tapping her paintbrush on the paper in front of her. A man comes in and asks if this is all the entertainment today. He doesn't look impressed and walks out.

Daphne is sobbing still, shivering, resonant of a child forced to go to school when all is not well. Gemma says that she has had a chest infection and that she is on antibiotics. 'Very cold,' says Daphne. She pushes herself up in the chair and slowly she leaves the room. She walks on a few paces and stumbles a bit. The second man that visited the activities room appears behind. 'Well I think they need to get us all out to the beach or something,' he says, wanting a change of scene.

She walks towards the main lounge. She sees one of the unit's carers who says, 'hello. Welcome back.' She invites Daphne to sit down. 'Oh I would,' says Daphne. 'You have a chill,' says the carer. The carer leaves the room and returns with a fleecy blanket and another larger one. She asks Daphne if she would like them. Daphne smiles, 'I would, yes please.' The carer places them over Daphne's legs, up to her waist. 'That might be nicer,' she says. 'It's cold.' 'It is,' says Daphne. 'Thank you very much.' The carer offers Daphne a cup of tea. Daphne puts her arms under the blankets and her body begins to relax. The carer returns with a cup of tea and places it on a table, which she pulls up next to Daphne. 'You are kind,' says Daphne, as if this is what she has been in need of all morning.

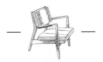

Dandelion, Daphne's unit, was empty. Given her bad cold the week before, you might have had a moment's panic that Daphne hadn't survived it. But this was not the case. The empty chairs were a sign that the home was having a deep clean. This meant moving the residents out of their usual routine and usual spaces. All of the residents from Dandelion group were mixed together with those from Cowslip.

It is full up in here, with residents sitting around tables in the dining area, many lined up near the television. This is a temporary camp for the homeless, an emergency refuge for those who have lost roofs and belongings. Some of the residents had lived through the Second World War and had been evacuated to other parts of the country as children. Was it all coming back to them? But the room was calm, the staff stoical, getting teas and biscuits and serving residents patiently. In fact, there was something of a team spirit among everyone, as if this temporary coming together was good for morale.

There's Daphne, huddled in one of the chairs, seated to the left of the kitchen. She looks as if she is being swallowed by the chair. She has on a large burgundy woollen cardigan around her shoulders on top of a pale green cardigan which is buttoned up around a striped linen shirt. She wears a black skirt with delicate circles on it and a pair of grey socks, tight just above the ankles. Daphne is not wearing her glasses. Her eyes are open, looking into the room, but it doesn't look as though she is focused on anything in particular. Gaynor, the woman who has recently had a stroke, has started to get up from the table. She begins to walk in Daphne's direction. Daphne pushes herself up in her chair and pulls the burgundy cardigan closer around her shoulders. She pushes both hands down on the hand rest, uncrosses her legs and makes to stand. When she stands she brushes a strand of hair from her face. She looks towards the door of the lounge and starts walking that way. Gaynor is also walking in that direction. She is just in front of Daphne.

They meet and stop. 'It is better to move,' Gaynor says, smiling at Daphne, as if she knows that this is not her place. Gaynor says something about carrying on and then lets out a laugh. Daphne laughs too. They are both making eye contact, engaged with one another. 'You are lovely,' says Daphne.

One of the cleaners walks past. She stops in front of the women. 'Hello, Daphne. Hello, Gaynor,' she says. The cleaner touches the side of Daphne's arm very gently, and Daphne smiles back. 'So kind,' she says.

So often touch brings comfort. Older people don't get enough of it. The two, in silence, stop as they get to the reception area. A senior member of staff walks past and stops to acknowledge both women, again using their first names and making eye contact. She smiles widely at both of them and explains that it is good to see them together. It is a brief moment of contact, a warm one.

'That was funny,' says Daphne. 'It is just like this, wobble wobble.' Gaynor smiles. She makes a sort of gobbledegook noise, shaking her head from side to side. Both Daphne and she start to laugh together. From afar the two women might look as if they are plotting something mischievous, in cahoots, but on closer inspection they are sharing experience, possibly struck by the absurd situation that they find themselves in.

They walk past the manager's office. Elaine is on the phone. The woman Daphne is with stops at a bright yellow bedroom door. It has a name on it. 'Joanne Gutheridge-Peeps'. Gaynor reads the name out loud. 'Joanne Gutheridge-Peeps. Look at that,' she says. 'What a bloody cheek.' Is Gaynor suggesting this is her room, or, worse still, her name – both place and identity taken from her?

The sun is shining through the double doors from the courtyard. It is very bright. 'This is lovely, this really is,' whispers Gaynor.

There is music coming from one of the rooms. The women walk past a lounge with several residents in, 'All there,' says Daphne, as if doing a head count in her mind. They continue walking into the room with the music 'Sweet Chariot'. The activities room is bright, as ever, with painted exotic animals and birds adorning the walls, as if we have entered the Amazon rainforest. There is a bright green balloon – a huge one – in the middle of the floor and a ball too. The chairs, bright red, orange or pale blue mock leather seats, with pine legs, are arranged in a circle. Despite its colour, it is always a cold room when no one is there: cut off, down the corridor, from daily life.

Gemma comes in with three other ladies, one using a zimmer frame, two walking unassisted. She invites them to sit in chairs opposite Daphne and Gaynor, who have taken up seats. A woman dressed in purple comes in and confidently sits herself down in a comfortable seat. Daphne is watching the movements and smiling.

A man in good physical shape comes in and says he is coming to see what it's all about. He sits down. Gemma comes back in with a man who is shuffling as he walks and another two women, one who is breathing heavily and is worried about falling. Gemma asks Daphne if she could move chairs so that this woman can have a chair closer to the entrance. 'Of course,' says Daphne. Gemma hands Gaynor the large green balloon. She holds it. Gemma leaves the room. Daphne is now seated in the chair central to the room, and is smiling as she looks around at each resident. The sprightly man, Dirk, gets up and leaves. It seems he has come to see Gemma. A woman next to Daphne says hello to her and says that she's lost about what they're doing. Who is leading the troupe?

Gemma returns; so does Dirk. Gemma stands in the middle of the circle. She asks Gaynor to pass the balloon. She is reluctant. Gemma asks her to hand it over and she will demonstrate. Gemma gently bats the balloon in the air in the direction of the woman who had difficulty walking to the room. She smiles, beams, and bops the balloon back in the air. It arrives opposite one of the residents who forces herself higher in her chair so she can reach the balloon and hit it again. Daphne is watching the balloon and singing to the background music at the same time. The balloon comes her way and she reaches forward and makes the balloon move forward back to Gemma. Gaynor has hit the balloon twice now, both times to the man who had shuffled in. He winks at her. Gemma explains that they will use their feet now doing football.

A heavier, leather ball moves around the room, and it is hard to take your eyes off all the feet. Some feet are tapping to the movement, some in position to kick, some just drooping down to the floor, relaxed. The ball goes to Daphne's feet and she brings both together and kicks the ball forward. Each time Gemma gets the ball, she democratically kicks it to those residents who haven't yet had a chance to do so. After some minutes, she takes the ball away.

She leaves the circle and changes the music and puts on a CD with a man talking in a very calm voice. 'Don't listen to him, though; all listen to me. Ok, so hands out in front of you and circle your wrists backwards and forwards.' Gemma demonstrates the moves. We might at this point imagine that the World Health Organisation's policy framework on active ageing (2002) had found its way into Winston Grove.

Daphne is happily engaging with the exercise routine. Every now and again someone loses track of what they are doing and Gemma says their name out loud, reminding them of the move. 'Ooh,' says one woman, rolling her eyes as if she has been caught out. One woman is moving forward in her chair, closing her eyes as if she might topple out of the chair. Gemma gets up and crouches down in front, gently pushing her back into her chair so that her back is supported. Daphne sees this. Just watching. She has put her hands inside the blanket which is resting on her legs.

'Pack up your troubles in your old kit bag and smile, smile, smile...' A stormy expression comes over Daphne's face. It is fleeting, momentary. Within seconds it disappears and she brings her hands back out of the blanket and raises them in the air, making rainfall motions with her fingertips.

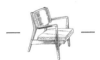

It was hard to predict what kind of a morning Daphne would have at Winston Grove. Gemma's timetable of activity seemed to be important to the life of the home, and also to Daphne's experience there. Sometimes, though, Daphne needed solitude. No activities were on hand this morning, the residents in Dandelion seemed to be cut off, either through their own withdrawal or some kind of organisational forgetting. Staff seemed short on the ground, the usual carers were not on shift, and the atmosphere slept as did the residents.

Daphne is seated in the main lounge. She is wearing a navy skirt, a striped linen shirt – purple and grey – and a grey mottled cardigan. She has slippers on. Her legs are crossed at the ankles and both of her arms are resting on armrests. Next to her a woman is sleeping heavily, sinking into the chair, a green blanket resting over her legs.

The permanent carer is seating residents one by one, folding napkins for each person as she does so. She puts salt and pepper on Daphne's table.

Daphne is seated opposite Gaynor. It is good to see her again. Daphne moves her napkin and puts it under her knife. Gaynor starts to talk about the days and the people and the work that is being done. She is poetic but words keep escaping her, whole sentences inchoate. Daphne looks at her and smiles, 'You are lovely,' she says.

Bridget is in the dining area, saying hello to each resident. She opens the curtains to bring some light in. The sun is shining brightly. Daphne grimaces. 'It is far too light,' she says. To account for everybody's needs is an ideal, but an unlikely reality.

The permanent carer is pouring out orange squash for each resident and placing it in front of them. She turns to ask the temporary carer, who has now come back, to start dishing up. Zalee, the temp, had been standing next to the trolley, waiting for further instruction as if her own authority has taken a temporary break. Bridget joins in to help, sensing that lunch is on a go-slow. There is a conversation about the woman with the bright light near her. Bridget asks her what food is going to be appropriate – soft food? She suggests that they give her chips to suck on for now. She bends down to the resident and says, smiling, 'well we just hope you won't choke.' And you wonder, not for the first time today, if some sadistic thought has just leaked out.

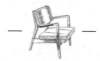

Daphne took little pleasure in an impromptu party the following week. She had not seen Benjamin that week and quite possibly there was an ache that prevented her from engaging with the life of the home.

Gemma is being followed by three walking residents. She puts on some music. Several residents are already in the lounge, one of whom is asleep and looks as though she is about to fall out of her chair. Gemma suggests to the carer, Diane, who is care planning, that perhaps she had better be moved. 'Help me then,' Diane says, perhaps irritated by the interruption. Diane gets up and together they adjust the woman's position.

Daphne walks into the middle of the lounge space where Dirk, who has followed Gemma, is now standing and batting a pink balloon in the air. One woman, who always looks down at the floor, is stepping from side to side, moving her hands to the beat of the music. Daphne comes in to stand with them and starts clapping. 'Roll out the Barrel,' she sings, smiling. Gaynor, who has been seated, gets up too and begins to join the dance, also singing at the top of her voice. The atmosphere is full of promise.

'Roll out the Barrel, we'll have a barrel of fun, Roll out the barrel...' Songs from wartime days fill the room. The four residents are dancing, all close to one another, singing, but at their own tempo. Daphne is pushing her arms out one at a time as if she is trumpeting; the woman who looks down is side-stepping; Dirk is standing still moving only his arms and Gaynor is clapping in a lively way.

Gemma asks Daphne to sit down next to Dirk. A balloon is thrown around a group of approximately twelve residents. Daphne smiles as she bats the balloon back to Gemma. Dirk tries to hit it too. Daphne is watching the balloon move between the residents. 'When Irish eyes are smiling,' she begins to sing in time. The balloon stops between Gaynor and Dirk. He bends forwards and tries to tap the balloon out of Gaynor's hand. 'That was disgusting, it was,' says Gaynor. He tries to bat the balloon out of her hand again. 'You are being too rough,' she says. Daphne clutches her hands together. Gaynor stands over Dirk, fearlessly. He pushes the balloon out of her hand, and now that her hands are free she pats him as hard as she can on his arm. 'Don't you do that again,' she says. Gaynor's recovery has been amazing.

Daphne stands up and pushes herself between man and woman, and walks into the middle of the room. Gaynor, buddying up, follows Daphne and together they start to dance. 'You are nice,' says Daphne.

A male carer walks in, saying hello to Gaynor. He holds her hands, dancing with her to the music. Ursula, a female carer, walks into the room and sees Daphne dancing alone and stands by her, mirroring her arm movements and marching as Daphne is. 'Fun,' she says. There is a party-like atmosphere in this part of the room where residents are dancing with staff.

Gemma puts three hoopla targets on the floor in front of residents who are seated. She is encouraging them to aim for the targets. A man slumped in his chair is nonetheless playing and has managed to get eight of ten rings on the targets. He is pleased with himself; the carers in the room are praising him. Dirk takes his turn next and doesn't do so well. 'You're not so good at that,' says the man in the chair, competitively.

'Let's get out of here now,' says Daphne, almost trying to reverse out of the room.

She walks towards the toilet area, stops for a minute, then doubles back towards the entrance and stands again next to a male carer also on the periphery of the room, uncertain about whether to engage. She looks agitated, repeating that she doesn't know what this is and what she is to do. 'This is life,' she says.

Daphne goes back to the toilet area, past a wall with objects from the 1940s dangling from it (certificates, gas marks, maps). She turns past a line of wheelchairs, some whole and some with parts missing. She stands in front of a toilet door, wide open. She peers into it. 'Well, there's no tower there, is there? You won't want to be here for that long,' she says. You wonder whether Daphne fears there is nothing stable here.

She looks back at the wheelchairs. 'I won't be doing that for them.' She goes back to where the music is in the lounge. She stands a moment peering in, a character very much on the periphery. 'Let's get out of here. It's a very silly world. I am sure they could do something about it.' Daphne takes a deep breath. 'It's all outside,' she says, as if she is talking about real life, about Benjamin, about where she wants to be.

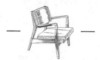

Daphne is now alone at Winston Grove; the promise of Benjamin's visits have ended with his unexpected death. Her way back to someone who accepted all her foibles was now a route closed off. The only diversion was Gemma, the deputy manager, someone, somewhere who understood the differences in tone between all of Daphne's 'Hey Hos'.

A walk is being organised. The carers offer up some names of residents who might like to go, and Gemma speaks with the men and women who have been selected. One woman is adamant that she wants to stay in. She asks Suki, who enthusiastically agrees. Daphne walks into the room where Gemma and another carer, Celia, are getting residents ready to go out.

'Their worlds don't understand my world; my world doesn't understand theirs,' says Daphne. 'They are too busy. They can't pay attention to you.' She begins to make this quivering, anxious noise again, holding her hands together tightly around her. You imagine Daphne is falling apart inside. She begins to stare at an empty chair, lost, while Celia is getting one woman ready. This woman doesn't have a coat in her bedroom and so Celia sacrifices hers for now. 'Is that okay?' The woman puts on the carer's coat and seems delighted. 'Oh well, very well then,' she says. 'How wonderful this is.'

'I think all I can do is sit down,' says Daphne. She goes to a chair, stands over it but doesn't sit down. She walks back towards the carer, Diane, who is now speaking with Suki who seems to have changed her mind about going out. Daphne is watching. 'Help me, help me,' she says in a quiet voice.

'What will I do then?' she asks. 'Well you are going out on Thursday,' says Diane to Daphne, but going out, we know, is for Benjamin's funeral. This is not for leisure. 'I want to come with you,' says Daphne to Diane.

'Well I am staying here with you, Daphne, and we can make some tea together and eat some custard creams.'

'Oh good,' says Daphne. 'I don't really know what to do. Can we help each other?' Daphne is clutching at people.

Diane agrees that they can and explains to Daphne that she can wait a few moments in the chair for her. Gemma explains that she could take someone else.

Gemma asks Daphne if she would like to come with her, for a coffee and a cake to the local shops. Daphne smiles, 'Oh yes please,' she says. 'Can my friend come?' she points at me. 'Do you think Daphne will be able to walk the whole way?' asks Gemma of Diane. 'I don't think so. I wouldn't risk it.'

'It's a funny old world,' says Daphne, waiting for someone to fetch her coat. She looks out into the room, watching the woman who is waiting in the wheelchair to go out.

Ursula comes in, offering Daphne a black coat with lining and big round buttons. Daphne slowly puts her left arm into the coat and then the right. Ursula begins to zip Daphne up, but it is a fiddle, 'Ouch,' says Daphne. Ursula says it is a little difficult, and starts to pull the buttons together instead. 'That's better,' says Daphne.

Ursula says she will try to fetch a scarf because it is so cold. She goes into the lounge and comes back with one and wraps it gently around Daphne. There is a wait in the reception area. The carer tucks the scarf into Daphne's coat. 'I don't know why they're all making me do these things. I just don't know why I can't do it myself. I don't want to be going out. I want to stay here. It's all I have,' and Daphne is right. Winston Grove is all she has now, stripped of her life and the people who made it hers.

Gemma comes out of the office, announces that 'we're off,' takes the woman in the wheelchair and the resident who looks down when she walks. A further temporary carer holds onto Daphne's arm. Bridget opens the doors, holding them ajar for everyone to leave.

Daphne feels the cold immediately. She begins to make ongoing quivering noises, as if she is freezing. The carer explains that it is cold but that it won't be a long walk. Daphne won't speak. She is making anxious noises. 'It's too chilly,' she says. 'Why are they doing this to me?' The outside, her outside, is intolerable to her now, persecutory. The high street and its cafes so far out of reach.

But then two small children go by on scooters. 'Look at these little loves,' says Daphne. She bends down to look at them, smiling. It seems that she might settle after all.

Another little boy on a bike goes by, and he looks so wobbly as if reminding Daphne of her own precariousness. 'Poor chap,' says Daphne. She continues making sounds as if she is going to cry. 'I don't know what is happening,' she says. 'And it's freezing.' A little girl in a buggy goes past and makes eye contact with Daphne, and this seems to offer comfort, 'Hello, sweetie,' says Daphne.

We walk up the road past a small school and then past a small theatre centre, coming to the cafe. The carer pushes the button on the door and Daphne, the carer, and Dirk enter. It is a lot warmer inside. 'That's better,' says Daphne. 'But what is this? What are we to do here?' The carer explains that she is going to get coffees and cakes for everyone. The carer walks Daphne and Dirk to the back of the room and finds a small table, with only two chairs. She invites them to take the two seats while she finds four other seats to accommodate everyone. Daphne is looking around her. 'There's a lot of women here. What's that screaming?' she hears some small children around the corner, looks at them. 'Poor children,' she says, imagining that they are in pain.

'There are our ladies,' she says, noticing Gemma come in with the woman in the wheelchair and the other woman who walks with her head down. Once everyone is seated, the carer asks everyone what they would like. 'That's four coffees, three hot chocolates.'

'I hope my sister will come here. But I am worried that she has too much on with her daughter,' says Daphne, anxiously.

The woman in the wheelchair reaches over and tries to pick up a napkin from the floor. Daphne offers it up. The woman is studying the words on the napkin. 'I don't know what I am supposed to do here,' says Daphne. The cakes and hot drinks arrive, and the carer cuts the cakes and hands pieces to each resident. Daphne takes her piece and begins to eat it. 'Very nice,' she says.

She is concentrating on eating. 'That's very good,' says Dirk, smiling. The resident who always looks down is putting her hands into the top of a creamy hot chocolate and licking her creamy fingers. Gemma offers her a piece of cake in a napkin and she begins eating the napkin too, unable to distinguish between that and the cake. Gemma hands her a fresh piece of cake. The lady looks up and starts laughing. Dirk starts laughing.

Daphne starts laughing too. 'Fun after all,' she says. 'This is life, really,' she says. She looks at the woman who is eating much of the cake. 'The children are happier. That's what it's all about. It's about the children, about happiness, about care…' Daphne stops and looks around her. 'There's a shortage of joy, shortage of men.'

She looks at the men and women sitting in the cafe, some on laptops, some women with children eating. 'I'm looking at that little girl,' says Daphne. 'It's funny because she is looking at me too.' Reminders of our own vulnerabilities. The little girl is not facing Daphne.

Looking at Daphne during these increasingly cold months was never just looking because she invited you in both to Winston Grove, and to her way of seeing life there. Closing the main door to Winston Grove and to Daphne's life was made harder knowing that Benjamin wouldn't be back the following week to take her out to the places she had once known and to see the children she so readily identified with. But I knew that in her mind she would find Benjamin and her sister Diane in other residents and staff there. And there was Gemma whom she knew was one of 'her ladies', and Gaynor, someone she might in the outside world have once called her friend.

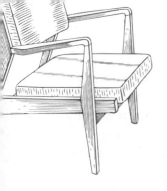

WHITTINGHALL

Unlike Winston Grove, you couldn't reach Whittinghall by public transport. There were no tube, train or bus links here. Along winding country roads, over bridges across the River Thames, past at least several stately homes, garden centres, and historic pubs serving home-cooked locally sourced food, Whittinghall could be found on the outskirts of a pretty village in Middle England. Close enough to commuter towns for workers in the City and far enough away for once weary Londoners to drop down to a slower pace, the surrounding areas of Whittinghall were in the main affluent, conservative, and very, very green.

Whittinghall was not close to shops, restaurants, art houses or businesses. It could be found to the right of small turning lined with several modern brick houses. Whittinghall was also a large brick contemporary home, large enough to accommodate many older people from the local area. The car park in front was spacious, spots always available for visitors and staff. An extensive landscaped garden went all the way around the house, and two imposing balconies at the front of the home could give residents the opportunity to watch the comings and goings. Being light and the beginning of summer, you might have expected to see some residents taking in the warmth of the sun, appreciating the woodland and fields in the distance.

Part of a private care home organisation, Whittinghall was able to provide a combination of residential, nursing, palliative, and specialist dementia care. The organisation, Wellbank Homes, prided itself, according to its promotional literature, on having its own dementia care policies. In recent times it had received several accolades. Whittinghall had been awarded a 'good' in its CQC inspection. Seemingly the home had had input from experts in the field of dementia care design: fabrics were warm and bespoke, carpets and wallpapers offered comfort and luxuriousness. Walking into Whittinghall was like walking into a four-star hotel. It made you want to sit down, have a coffee and read the paper. Smells of urine, bodies, disinfectant were absent. Residents were not conspicuous at reception and so there were just some small telling signs that alerted you to the true purpose of the building you were in: photographs of older people playing a quiz, a notice about an upcoming relatives' meeting, and the many signs – the signs on toilets, clear and in bright yellow, the signs for corridors, categorising spaces, and memory boxes or photographs on the front of bedroom doors. These were the dementia-friendly signs that any good home would have. They were also the acceptable faces of frailty – degrees of frailty. Instead of reading 'nursing', 'dementia' or 'palliative', units were given names that might be found on any house or street instead: 'Huntside', 'Appleyard', 'Berryhill'.

There was a receptionist who greeted visitors on arrival, directed them to the signing-in book and called upon a member of staff, or the manager, Amy, to show them in and around. This was an efficiency that Winston Grove was very much without.

Nancy appears at reception and says hello to the receptionist. She smiles a warm smile, and takes me around the corner. To the right is a large dining room, with a man pushing a trolley, dressed in blacks and whites like a waiter. Tables are dressed with coloured napkins, tablecloths, table mats, a vase of flowers on each. No cutting corners here. 'Our unit is elderly frail, although we have lots of dementia too,' Nancy says, coming out of the lift, entering 'Huntside'. In this unit, professional roles are clear, colour coded by uniforms: nursing staff in a range of blues, care workers in light and dark green trousers, activity assistants in brown top and bottom combos, and waiting staff in black and whites. A hairdresser in her own clothes occupies the hair salon at different times of the week and occasionally a visiting physiotherapist, vicar or chaplain will come by.

Dorothy is sitting in her wheelchair next to a table opposite the nurses' station. A young nurse is behind the station, filling out paperwork. Nancy stoops down to Dorothy and gently touches her arm. A half-smile forms on Dorothy's lips. 'Remember Esther has come to visit us Dorothy,' continues Nancy. 'She's just come up from downstairs.' An episode of upstairs, downstairs; a need to compartmentalise.

'Very nice,' says Dorothy. 'Very nice.'

'You have to speak loud. Her hearing is...' says Nancy, assuming Dorothy can't hear and that I will be talking a lot.

Dorothy either doesn't hear or ignores it. Nancy is still stooped down, her upper body just above Dorothy's feet, which are resting on the footrests of the wheelchair. Nancy is looking up at Dorothy, as if she is a dutiful servant to a formidable woman, yet she continues to speak as if Dorothy is not there.

'Dorothy has been here since Autumn,' says Nancy, still crouched down. 'She is very attached to me now. She calls me "Wendy" and asks after me when I leave the room. Sometimes she pushes her foot down in her wheelchair to move to come and find me, don't you, Dorothy?' Nancy says, now trying to engage her charge. Dorothy doesn't say anything, failing to provide any supporting evidence. She has both hands placed on the wheelchair armrests, staring towards Nancy.

Dorothy flinches momentarily as Nancy touches her purple-slippered toes. 'Sorry,' says Nancy, 'if that hurt.'

'Tues----day,' says Dorothy, noticing a sign for today placed on the wall of the nurses' station.

'We've put that there,' says Nancy, 'because some of the residents sometimes call out Saturday when it isn't.' Perhaps it's always the weekend, time to go out, to do something different, hook up with relatives, take in a show...?

Dorothy doesn't seem bothered that Nancy is talking about her, and the other residents, as if she is not there. Nancy goes on to explain some of the details of Dorothy's life. Dorothy has a daughter, three grandchildren. 'She doesn't come that much,' says Nancy about the daughter. 'Wendy isn't her daughter,' says Nancy. 'We don't know who Wendy is. I think it's just a name she calls me.' This sounds like a mystery.

Dorothy looks towards both of us but sort of stares through us then she takes a deep breath, bends her head down onto her chest, as if she has been winded momentarily. It is hard to know the significance of this moment. The silence – what do we put in the silence, in the gaps? Something to ponder momentarily before we carry on with our visit at Whittinghall.

'We just don't know who Wendy is. We have asked friends and family. No one knows. She also calls one of the men "Tony" but none of us know who that is either. You've got a good friend Letty, haven't you, Dorothy?' On hearing Letty's name, Dorothy looks up and makes eye contact with Nancy and smiles. There is comfort in this name, this echo from a friendly past.

'You used to look after animals, didn't you?' asks Nancy of Dorothy. Nancy is filling in pieces of the story that seem as though they will never come from Dorothy alone, factual details, filling in the gaps in Dorothy's existence, making her come to life. Again Dorothy makes eye contact. 'I did, some time ago.' 'Yes,' says Nancy, 'that's what Letty told me when she came, and that you used to have dogs, horses, I think.' Letty had been to the home to see her old friend once. Letty had not come since. She was very far away and old too. You wondered whether Letty would ever make it again.

'Tueeess-day,' says Dorothy.

'Yes it is Tuesday,' says Nancy.

'It's not Tuesday.'

'Oh it is,' says Nancy. This is the kind of minor conflict that happens between people, the kind of conflict mothers and children might have. Some can be written off; some can't. Some battles are worth fighting; others not. This is one dispute which will benefit no one.

'Dorothy's from somewhere in Scotland originally,' Nancy says. 'Aren't you?'

Dorothy gives no response.

Sensing a rejection, or just the sheer hard work of engagement, Nancy explains that she has to go and see some other residents to make sure they are okay. Dorothy is now in the corridor alone apart from the nurse who is doing the paperwork behind the station.

A chaplain enters, asking for a resident. The nurse gets up and shows him towards a bedroom. 'Well I doubt he has moved,' says the visitor. The nurse explains that he could have gone to the activities, as if correcting the chaplain on the possibility of movement in the home.

Dorothy is watching all this, quizzically.

Dorothy puts her head back into her hands again. 'Where have they all gone?' she says staring into empty space.

Nancy walks back into the corridor, on cue, asking Dorothy if she is okay. Dorothy nods and follows Nancy with her eyes then looks back at the nurses' station wall. 'Tuesday,' she says.

Nancy goes to get several cups of tea. Dorothy rests one hand on top of the other and examines her fingernails momentarily. She stares at the wall opposite her.

Nancy returns with two cups of tea, one in a two-handled beaker for Dorothy. She places the tea down in front of me and hands the beaker to Dorothy, explaining that it is hot. 'Too hot,' says Dorothy, ushering Nancy to place it down next to her. Nancy notices a male member of staff in the distance and says that Dorothy does not like men; she says that they are 'horrible'.

'Tuesday,' says Dorothy. You might begin to think that this piece of signage is like a security blanket for Dorothy; an attachment object, a strange comfort, something that situates her and makes her life real. But this is only supposition.

A woman in a black tee shirt goes past and Dorothy looks at her. The woman stops and says, 'hello Dorothy.' Her face lights up. 'Hello,' she says. 'You'll be coming to have your hair done later today.' This is the hairdresser. 'Oh,' says Dorothy, happily.

'Dorothy loves having her hair done,' says Nancy. There are two hairdressers and they cover all the days of the week for all the residents. This is a good service.

Nancy and the hairdresser have a brief chat about whom the hairdresser should see first. Nancy follows the hairdresser into the hairdressing suite. Dorothy sits on, moving her feet slightly then stopping. She pays no attention to her tea or juice next to her.

Nancy returns and bends down next to Dorothy, facing her. 'Do you want your hair done?' Dorothy shakes her head, 'Not now, no. Maybe later.' Nancy smiles at Dorothy. 'Oh but you love it, don't you, and it'll be nice for you, it will.'

'Not yet, though,' says Dorothy calmly. Perhaps moving would take up a lot of energy.

'You will feel better when you have had it done though.' This might take the pressure off Nancy, who may feel the weight of being observed.

'Ok then, whatever you think,' says Dorothy, trusting her keyworker.

Nancy bends further down, gently placing Dorothy's feet in the wheelchair footrests. She explains what she is doing and then moves behind Dorothy and begins to push her towards the hairdressing suite. The hairdresser is in place and welcomes Dorothy in. She explains that she will put her hair in rollers today. The radio is on in the background, quietly. There are two mirrors in the suite, and two seats with sinks for the residents. Nancy pushes Dorothy towards a sink and helps the hairdresser put the towels around Dorothy's back. The hairdresser places a wet proof cover around Dorothy and the hairdresser tells her that she will check the water is warm enough. A lot of care goes into this procedure. Nancy asks Dorothy to begin to move forward and put her chin down so that her head will be over the sink as far as possible. Nancy is gently applying pressure to Dorothy's back, which is stiff and unbending. She makes no complaints.

The hairdresser starts to wet Dorothy's hair with the shower head and then applies shampoo. All the while Nancy is behind Dorothy, standing with her and placing a firm hand on her back. Dorothy makes no noises. Once the wash and rinse is finished, the hairdresser dries Dorothy's hair and takes a towel edge and wipes her eyes with it. Dorothy sits upright and notices herself in the mirror and keeps on looking at herself, without expression. Does she recognise herself now, aged?

The hairdresser is taking off the towels but Dorothy holds onto one. 'You want to keep that one, Dorothy?' says the hairdresser, letting her hold onto it.

Nancy leaves. The hairdresser begins to get the box of rollers and Dorothy sits perfectly still, her hands resting on the top of the sink. An activities worker, in brown, walks in and pushes her face round the side of the hairdresser so that she can say hello to Dorothy. 'You gonna have nice clean hair now? That's nice.' 'Um,' says Dorothy, baffled by this appearance. The carer picks up Dorothy's hands and looks at her fingernails. 'They so nice now, aren't they? I do like them, they are better than mine,' she says. 'And you got nice clean hair now, so lovely.' She walks away, one-way conversation over.

Nancy comes back in and stands with a thick comb in her hand. She watches the hairdresser doing Dorothy's hair and asks when she will have a perm next. They agree on a fortnight.

This morning had been a busy one for Dorothy. She had received a visitor, Nancy had found the time to be by her side during most of that hour, and there'd been a visit to the hairdressers. In all that time, Dorothy had said only a few words and repeated some; her body itself had not moved a great deal, and there had been no laughter. Time seemed to have ticked on slowly. Although things were happening, you imagined them happening again in the same way, at the same time. Each time Dorothy called out 'Tuesday' you had a sense that she had been here before; watching her left you with a heaviness of being, the experience of eternal recurrence, of Tuesday in the corridor.

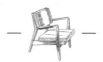

Familiarity is important in dementia care. Consistent staff members, consistent environments, consistent touch and tone. There was no doubt that it was consistent at Whittinghall. Dorothy took up the same place in the home each week, and Nancy was almost always on shift. When Nancy wasn't there other members of the team struggled to fill her absence, as we shall see today. Nancy has taken a week's holiday with friends, as young people do. A scheduled break, but one that seems unexpected for Dorothy.

Dorothy is in the corridor, opposite the nurses' station. Another woman in a wheelchair is parked next to her. A senior male carer in a white coat is behind the station; another carer to his side, filling out a form. Dorothy is sleepy. The carer says that she can move Dorothy into the lounge. She goes behind Dorothy and begins wheeling her into the lounge. No words are exchanged. Dorothy is pushed past the dining tables, a grand piano with a giant lion on top to her left, and a row of sofas. This is where Dorothy stops. There is no one in the lounge apart from a woman in a wheelchair closer to the television, a fashion show playing.

Dorothy looks towards the television, shaking her head, then looks down to her stomach. The carer returns with orange juice in a glass, putting it in front of Dorothy. 'You can talk to Dorothy if you want,' she says. This injunction to speak comes as a surprise.

Dorothy looks at her hands, she has light pink nail polish on. She brings both hands down to her sides and pulls her top down a little. She is wearing a lime green cardigan over a mint and white, spotty collared t-shirt, with green trousers. Her colours are co-ordinated, and your mind flits back to the fashion show on the television. On her feet are burgundy slippers. She pushes herself up in her chair a little, looking down at her feet then slouches back in the wheelchair. She looks out of the window and for a while, and just keeps staring at the trees blowing in the wind. She turns to the television, keeps her focus for a few minutes, then shakes her head.

The carer walks back into the room and peels a banana in front of Dorothy. 'She likes bananas,' says the carer. 'She didn't have much breakfast. Oh this banana is bruised,' she says, taking it away. As she throws the banana in the bin, she says from behind, 'With a banana she might speak to you. Sugar.' Commentary seems to go on around Dorothy as if she is not there. Double-triple isolations. Bananas… animals performing tricks, come to mind, but this is harsh.

She brings back another banana, hands it to Dorothy who immediately begins eating very slowly. She takes a bite then chews slowly, studying what is left. Dorothy peels the banana as far down as possible and eats the small hardened bit that is left. She turns and quietly hands me the skin. I take it in my hands and she looks at the banana skin there. Like a transitional object, this movement between seems to have conferred some kind of meaning, but it is unclear what.

She turns back to the television. 'I don't know what that is.' Has the sugar brought on speech? Or the sharing of the skin? 'I don't know,' she says.

Dorothy looks outside towards the trees. 'Windy, windy, windy.' She puts her head down in her right hand and stays there for some minutes, unmoving.

'I don't know where I am.' Making an attempt at connection and reassurance, I utter the factual detail of where she is. It doesn't help. She shakes her head, as if to say no. Perhaps this doesn't ring true. Is Dorothy somewhere else?

An activities assistant comes in with two boxes and starts counting library books in the corner of the room. Another activities assistant comes in and there is some discussion about lost library books. In Whittinghall, as in other care homes, people and things get lost. Physically or psychically lost or forgotten.

The first assistant starts removing the books from the bookshelves; the second talks to the woman watching television. She asks her how she is, how her daughter is. Sensing the need for holding and touch, the activities assistant puts her arm around her momentarily. The woman's feet aren't in the right place on the wheelchair. 'Let's move you,' she says, 'before you lose a leg.' Something else is out of place.

Dorothy has been watching, and looks down at her own feet. She notices that a piece of material from the wheelchair footrest is in front of her feet. 'I'll be fine, fine, fine,' she says.

Behind Dorothy two men in black waistcoats and dicky bows have come into the room with a drinks trolley. They are chatting. Dorothy says there's too much noise behind her. The activities assistant joins in the chat, telling them about her new tattoo. Dorothy tries to turn her head but she cannot twist it around enough to see what is going on. She makes another effort to turn her head, but gives up. When she looks up she has tears in her eyes.

The activities assistant with the tattoo tries to engage Dorothy in a conversation about the inking. She shows Dorothy an underwater scene on her leg. Dorothy shakes her head as if she is revolted by it, screwing up her face. 'Dorothy doesn't like it at all.' The assistant walks away. Mutual rejection.

'Where are they?' asks Dorothy. She looks tearful again.

A man with a black and white bandana enters the room with a hot food trolley, followed by one of the men in dicky bows, and a nurse. The activities assistant with the books walks back in with another male carer, who is trying to help her find two lost books.

An older woman, a resident, walks in, sitting herself at the dinner table. She waits alone for some time. Another carer comes in, pushing a lady in a wheelchair to the table. The books still haven't been found. There is a discussion about the library penalising them.

The carer explains to the woman watching television that it is lunchtime, so she moves her to the table with the other two women. There is a threesome around the table now. Dorothy notices that this carer is back in the room and tries to get her attention. Now four members of staff are by the trolley in the kitchenette, discussing who is having what. Dorothy lets out a noise and raises her hand, the thumb closing in on the fingers and touching them, making a sort of birdlike shape. In Whittinghall's promotional blurb, these kitchenettes are important spaces – informal ones – where residents can come together, relax, socialise and share tea. Today the enhanced communal living is enjoyed by the members of staff.

The carer asks me if it's alright to move Dorothy for lunch. 'Lunch, lunch, lunch.' Thankfully Dorothy speaks for herself. The carer starts pushing her to the table.

Dorothy, alone at the table, is given a glass of orange juice by a nurse. She makes a noise as if trying to get someone's attention but nobody notices. She pulls her face back as if to make a scream but nothing comes out. Edvard Munch understood this kind of crippling angst. Tears come to Dorothy's eyes. She pushes the orange juice away, rejecting and rejected.

The waiter takes a bowl of tomato soup over to Dorothy. That too, she pushes off the tablemat. There is some conversation behind about me having lunch, too, a strategy to help Dorothy to eat. The carer asks me if I could join her and have some soup and she might copy me, filling in for Nancy, her attachment?

Dorothy shows no interest in eating.

The activities assistant with the books arrives next to Dorothy. 'I've got your new slippers here.' Dorothy shakes her head. The assistant starts to move Dorothy backwards from the table, takes the slippers out to show her. Dorothy puts her head in her hands. 'Let's try them on to make sure they fit,' she says. She removes Dorothy's old slippers and puts the new ones on. Dorothy looks down as this happens. 'They fit,' says the assistant excitedly, a pantomime moment. Dorothy looks dejected, despite the new footwear. 'You're missing your friend, aren't you?' She turns to me. 'She never speaks when Nancy is away. She'll be like this until she's back next Tuesday.' You wonder whether this is because no one else is listening.

Dorothy is not interested in mirroring me. Mothers, or mother figures, aren't so easily replaced. The waiter takes the soup in a bowl, replacing it with soup in a sippy cup. Dorothy shakes her head. She looks tearful, as if no one recognises her plight.

A little boy with his mother, visiting grandfather you imagine, comes into the dining room and sits down. They all have lunch, a family of three generations. Dorothy is taken with the little boy and smiles. 'Lovely, lovely, lovely,' she says, 'little boy.' She begins to bend her fingers to wave at him. He waves back. She smiles.

What Dorothy sees in this little boy we can only imagine, something of her youth, of a time when she was looked after and had family? Whatever it is, the little boy sees Dorothy and responds to her reaching out in a way that the Whittinghall team haven't managed to do today in Nancy's absence. We shall see that Dorothy sometimes rejects, and sometimes is rejected; she is one of those residents with whom any of us might find it tricky to relate. Getting to know Dorothy demands patience and perseverance because at times she builds walls that are impermeable... although her walls might well be a reflection of the walls that house her too.

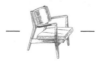

Two weeks passed: school holidays had interrupted the visits. Amy, the manager of the home, knew this but Nancy did not. With her week's holiday and my break of a fortnight, this meant that three weeks had elapsed before I had seen Dorothy and Nancy together again. Nancy was a little confused to see me.

Nancy is walking towards the lift with her young colleagues, and tries to place me in her mind. She says that she thought she hadn't seen me for a while. The message given to her boss, Amy, didn't seem to have been relayed. Dorothy was unlikely to have been reminded about the break in visits too. Me: another lost object.

Nancy says that Dorothy hasn't been eating well; she's been agitated recently. She'd been told Dorothy had missed her while she was on holiday and that she had barely talked. On her return, Dorothy had clung to Nancy adhesively.

A male nurse and carer are sitting in the nurses' station. Dorothy is sitting opposite the station, as she was before the break. She looks low. Nancy walks up to her and says hello.

Dorothy puts her head up. 'Hello…' She looks towards Nancy. 'Wendy, Wendy, Wendy,' she says three times.

Nancy asks if any tea or coffee is needed. 'Tea,' says Dorothy. She watches intently, eyes glued, as Nancy walks away to the kitchen area.

A young girl dressed in black trousers and a black waistcoat with a white shirt walks past with a trolley. 'Dorothy will,' says the girl about the biscuits on her trolley: a foregone conclusion. She offers the plate to Dorothy who looks at the tray of biscuits and chooses two malt biscuits. 'Oh, two,' says the waitress. 'Of course.' Dorothy smiles, puts one biscuit down on the table to her left and takes a bite of the other. She stops there, and puts the biscuit on the side of her wheelchair arm.

She notices some crumbs have fallen on her gilet cardigan and her brown trousers, and starts to flick them off. A carer gets up from the nurses' station and walks away, explaining to Nancy that she is taking a break. Breaks don't seem hard to come by at Whittinghall.

Nancy returns with tea for Dorothy in a two-handled beaker. Dorothy touches the tea and shakes her head again as if to say it is too hot. 'You don't want the tea yet,' says Nancy. 'Too hot.' 'Um,' says Dorothy, chewing her biscuit.

She notices more crumbs fall and brushes them away. She finishes chewing her biscuit and puts her head and face back into her right hand, staying there for some minutes. 'What's wrong?' Nancy asks Dorothy, rubbing her left arm as she asks the question. Dorothy looks up, 'Nothing's wrong, wrong, wrong.'

Nancy says that Dorothy has been agitated recently and shows me with her feet how Dorothy was trying to follow her on her wheelchair, almost tipping herself up. Perhaps being parted during the break was too much. Dorothy is looking towards the nurses' station. The girl with the biscuits returns. Nancy asks her to stop for Dorothy. 'She has had two already.'

'It doesn't matter,' says Nancy.

'No, it doesn't to me. I've got loads of biscuits here,' says the girl. She presents Dorothy with the tray and Dorothy takes a chocolate biscuit. 'Thank you,' she says. Sugar, again.

Dorothy puts the chocolate biscuit on the table besides her. Nancy offers up the tea but Dorothy declines. Nancy picks up a glass with a little bit of orange juice left in it. She offers this to Dorothy. Dorothy meets Nancy's eyes and accepts the orange juice.

A man is calling out 'Help.' It's impossible to isolate where the calls are coming from unless you know him. It sounds like a moan. Perhaps a bedroom opposite the nurses' station. He shouts out again, this time a little more forcefully. The nurse at the station does not move. He calls out again. There is also a man in the corridor and a girl dressed in jeans, who might be a member of staff out of uniform, both talking to an activities co-ordinator. The man calls out again. No one goes to him. He stops calling.

Nancy offers to take a group of residents outside on the balcony if the weather is good, and explains that she would try to take Dorothy. She notices Dorothy is sleepy again and says that while Dorothy sleeps she talks non-stop. You imagine her watching Dorothy sleeping and chattering away, amazed that Dorothy is able to speak so much in sleep. Everything, everything she's held in.

One of the domestic staff walks past. Dorothy has woken up, and is watching him. 'He's weird,' she says. 'No he's not,' Nancy corrects her. Dorothy puts her head down, closing her eyes again. Nancy says that Dorothy's daughter came in last week with the grandchildren.

The activities assistant and the girl out of uniform walk towards Nancy. There is some conversation with the girl in the jeans about another member of staff not coming back, and another who is non-committal. The girl in jeans is the senior nurse in Huntside. Staffing woes are brought to her attention.

Nancy returns to where Dorothy is sitting, and talks about her job. She works from eight in the morning to eight at night, five days a week.

She is glad she gets her weekends off. Staffing isn't usually a problem in this unit; there are six permanent staff who have been working in the unit consistently from three to ten years. This is good.

'She is so sleepy because of this medication. She has two each day and then she is gone,' says Nancy.

Studies indicate that ninety per cent of people with dementia experience behavioural and psychological symptoms related to their condition, such as agitation, loss of inhibition, and aggression. However, people with dementia are often inappropriately prescribed anti-psychotic drugs to reduce behavioural and psychological symptoms. These are known to have serious side effects, and, though there can be a moderate benefit, the drugs do not address any underlying causes. Rather, they might be used as a sort of general tranquiliser, silencing people from expression. We might be able to see some of the underlying causes for Dorothy. One Department of Health study noted that, out of 180,000 prescriptions for people with dementia, 140,000 are inappropriate. There is a nine-fold risk of stroke in the first four weeks (Kleijer et al, 2009) and a near doubling in the risk of mortality (Food and Drug Administration, 2005). A national priority since the *National Dementia Strategy* (DoH, 2009) has been to reduce the prescription of anti-psychotics for people with dementia. There has been a call for a greater emphasis on holistic treatments of care for people with dementia expressing behavioural and psychological symptoms.

Whether Dorothy was being given anti-psychotic drugs and being sedated these few weeks was unknown, but it was clear from Nancy's accounts that Dorothy had been more troublesome in the home recently and that this was an ongoing issue. Would an observer note something of use, or simply provide extra company? It seemed clear that Dorothy often needed someone close by.

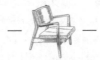

Summer continued. Often the weather was beautiful, the sun piercing through the swaying of leaves in this green country. Boats could be seen on the River Thames, with couples picnicking on open roofs, cafes full of diners outside, spilling onto cobbled pavements in the towns all around

Whittinghall. And in the home itself trips were being arranged for the residents, to make sure the summer months were enjoyed. Outside, people were in sandals and flip-flops, shorts and tee shirts. Inside Whittinghall, the young staff team continued to wear their uniforms and thick black shoes; residents continued to wear cardigans on top of blouses, jumpers on top of shirts, the changing of seasons and temperatures unnoticed indoors.

Nancy is at reception. Dorothy is more alert today, still sitting in the corridor. The male senior carer is sitting behind the nurses' station. A carer with dark glistening hair is looking for files there.

Nancy walks up to Dorothy, gently touching her arm. 'My new friend,' says Dorothy looking at me. Impressions were being made. This made it all the more difficult to think that her medication might at times stun her into emotional and social numbness.

'That's right,' she says. She looks at me, smiling. A red purse, mine, is on the table. 'What's that?' she says. 'What's that?'

'That's ok, that's ok, that's ok,' she says, looking at it. Inside are pictures of my children, and Nancy offers them up as a way of connecting. She knows Dorothy has always loved small children. Dorothy looks at them, smiling but unsure. They aren't hers.

Dorothy turns to the table and picks up a custard cream, and starts chewing it. A few crumbs spill onto her lime green jumper and, ever fastidious, she wipes them off with both hands. She pulls her jumper down ever so slightly into a straight line, ordering herself.

A 'waiter', pushing a trolley, walks past. 'There he is, there he is, there he is.' Dorothy knows the drill.

The young man takes a two-handled beaker and pours Dorothy a tea. Nancy takes it, handing it to Dorothy, explaining it isn't too hot. Nancy has got a swivel chair from behind the nurses' station and is sitting on it, very close to Dorothy now.

Dorothy takes the tea, sips a little. 'Not too hot, not too hot. You have some,' she says to Nancy. Nancy takes the beaker and makes out that she is sipping it. Dorothy takes great pleasure in this moment's sharing, which is something of a ritual. Dorothy likes giving to Nancy; she likes the mirroring.

Nancy asks the man with the trolley if she could have another biscuit for Dorothy. He passes Dorothy a plate and she takes another custard cream. A carer walks past. 'There's another one,' says Dorothy. Nancy shakes her head, and explains, 'Coloured skin. She says it about everyone who is black but at least she doesn't shout it out loud.' At this point, though Dorothy's noticing seems neutral rather than discriminatory, the diverse staff teams found in care homes can lead to racial tensions. While it is hard to find statistics relating to diversity in care homes, the Social Care Institute of Excellence (SCIE) recognises that dignity in care (2006)[12] is vital. Dignity for care workers forms an important component of this. SCIE points out that training and awareness-raising is crucial in ironing out the negative effects of cultural and racial differences between care workers and those in their charge. The impact of multicultural populations housed in one relatively small space, where needs are often already high, is often overlooked by policy-makers. Another taboo issue, along with death, dependency, and sexuality.

Dorothy notices a sign on the nurses' station, 'Thursday,' she says, 'Thursday, Thursday.'

'Yes,' says Nancy, 'it is Thursday.'

Dorothy was very agitated yesterday. Nancy puts it down to her not being there on weekends. Dorothy's daughter has said that Nancy had better not leave before Dorothy dies. Nancy says she couldn't bear to be there when Dorothy goes because she has got so close to her. Interestingly, Nancy is thinking of a time without Dorothy; it is in her mind. The burden on Nancy is great; as if she is responsible for Dorothy's psychic survival. She is talking about Dorothy's death while she is alive, right next to her. In some ways, in some moments, it is as if Dorothy is already dead.

Nancy pushes herself forward on the swivel chair and hands Dorothy the orange juice. Dorothy takes a sip. 'You love orange juice, don't you?' Dorothy puts the juice down and Nancy offers her the tea now. Dorothy hands Nancy the tea, 'For you, for you,' she says. Nancy takes it, pretending to sip from it. She hands it back to Dorothy who takes a sip. These instances of feeding are full of care, there is no doubt. But you can't help reflecting on the absence of psychic nourishment at Whittinghall.

At lunch Nancy has to eat what Dorothy is eating, but the other day it was salmon and Nancy just couldn't do it; she was repelled by the salmon. Or by the closeness. Perhaps both.

---

12 http://www.scie.org.uk/publications/guides/guide15/index.asp

A man walks past and Dorothy pulls a face. 'She doesn't like men,' says Nancy. For Nancy, Dorothy expresses several prejudices. Dorothy is perhaps considered hostile.

Nancy pushes herself close to Dorothy and asks her if she wants to go outside, explaining that it is hot and the trees look breezy. There might be cars outside, too. Dorothy always looks for a green car, her daughter's. But what if it isn't there? Hopes dashed. 'No, that's all right, that's all right, that's all right, no.' Dorothy smiles.

A man in a brown top walks past in the corridor with a hanger full of clothes. Dorothy laughs, 'Look at all those clothes, those clothes, those clothes.' It is a funny sight, like a shop-on-legs.

In the lounge behind Dorothy a word puzzle game is taking place with three residents and an activities assistant.

The man with the tea goes past again and Nancy stops him. Nancy asks for a chocolate biscuit. He gives her two. Nancy passes them to Dorothy. 'Only one, only one, only one,' she says. 'For you, for you, for you,' says Dorothy, holding one out to Nancy. 'Thank you,' she says, touched.

A man in his fifties walks in, a young-looking man, someone out of place in these corridors for the elderly. 'Where's my daughter?' Perhaps he has early onset dementia. Nancy and the man have a conversation. Dorothy considers him to be her son, but as far as we know she has never had one. 'That's your friend, isn't it?' asks Nancy.

'That's right, that's right, that's right,' says Dorothy, looking at him and smiling.

Dorothy tips her head down and begins to close her eyes. This has been a busy morning, and Dorothy has had enough.

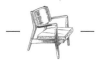

Dorothy was often sleepy and showed very little of the reported agitation when I saw her. Whether it was because she had had medication that made her drowsy earlier in the shift, or because waiting for 'Wendy' was so painful that only cutting off made her stay at Whittinghall bearable, it was impossible to know. Today, though, Dorothy was wide awake.

Nancy is dealing with files in the nurses' station. 'Oh good,' says Nancy to me. 'You can look after her.' The role of observer morphs into companion, carer, befriender. Dorothy is abruptly handed over.

Dorothy has pushed her torso upright in her wheelchair, pushing her feet onto the ground – they are out of her footrests – and she is trying to move the chair over to the nurses' station, to get closer to Nancy. This is the agitation. Her feet are behind the back of the footrests and she is pushing down on the floor, forcing the chair to move. This looks like a contorted manoeuvre for old, inflexible feet. 'Wendy, Wendy, Wendy,' she shouts, as if trying to hammer a nail into a plank that keeps on shifting. I explain that Wendy is just there. Dorothy bats into the air with one hand, as if to push my face out of the way. Dorothy is focused, determined, and angry.

'See,' says Nancy. 'She's been agitated today. Too much going on.'

Another carer appears, moving in to the nurses' station, also filling in forms. An atmosphere of preoccupation.

'Wendy, Wendy, Wendy,' shouts Dorothy, still pushing herself forward. She wants someone, something.

It is hard not to act. Dorothy shakes her head. My arm reaches out as if to settle her. Nancy comes out of the nurses' station. She asks Dorothy where she is going. 'There you are, there you are, there you are,' says Dorothy.

Nancy gets behind Dorothy, returns the chair, with Dorothy in it, back to the original position. The brakes are on. Dorothy starts moving her feet again. Nancy asks Dorothy to sit still for a moment. Nancy goes back into the nurses' station. This isn't what Dorothy wants.

'Wendy, Wendy, Wendy,' she shouts. Louder, louder, louder. She raises her hand into the air and makes that bird-like beak shape with it. 'What am I doing, doing, doing?' she says. Nancy doesn't answer; nor does the other carer. Dorothy shakes her head, putting her face in her hands. 'Don't know what I'm doing, doing, doing.' Nancy is busy filling in forms, not noticing what Dorothy is saying. Dorothy looks back down and puts her head in her hands. Watching this, you might be reminded of a harassed mother avoiding the interruptions of her demanding toddler. You might be reminded of Baraitser's (2009) work on interruptions and psychic crises. And you'll also feel just how much Dorothy needs someone.

The hairdresser comes out of the salon. 'Ridiculous,' she says, rattled. She walks past the nurses' station, mumbling something, and then walks back. 'I'm at the end of my tether.' This is a rare scene in Whittinghall; emotions – frustrated, angry ones – are leaking out, making a mess.

'Do you want me to get her?' says Nancy, calling after the hairdresser.

'Wendy, Wendy, Wendy,' shouts Dorothy. She starts forcing her chair to move again, by pressing both feet down to the ground again, one after the other.

The hairdresser is shouting something from the salon; Nancy is trying to have a conversation with her as she walks over to Dorothy. Dorothy has her hand in the air again, beaklike, as if trying to get Nancy's attention, trying to be fed. Nancy takes her chair and sits it in front of Dorothy with her file. Dorothy settles back down into her seat. 'That's better, is it?' Nancy knows Dorothy wants her close by, but it doesn't make it any easier.

'What you doing, doing, doing?' Dorothy asks Nancy, as the young woman starts opening her file on her knees again and filling in forms. Both a secure base and a busy worker.

'Doing work,' says Nancy.

'It's Thursday, Thursday, Thursday,' says Dorothy, as if holding on tightly to external reality.

'Yes it is,' says Nancy; she giggles while writing her notes. This was the wrong move.

'What are you laughing at, laughing at? It's not funny, funny, funny,' she says, frowning.

The hairdresser comes out of the salon.

'I can go and get her,' says Nancy who gets up, moving towards the hairdresser. Dorothy follows Nancy with her eyes and shakes her head.

'Wendy, Wendy, Wendy,' shouts Dorothy.

'Everyone's Wendy,' says another young male carer, contemptuously, walking past. 'There he is, there he is, there he is,' says Dorothy, scornfully.

The nurse, who oversees Huntside, walks into the station.

'Wendy, Wendy, Wendy,' shouts Dorothy. No one is responding. Dorothy starts pushing herself up again from her chair and moving it towards the nurses' station. 'My hair done, my hair, my hair,' she shouts. No one is watching Dorothy who begins to look unstable in the chair. The nurse notices. 'Yes you will have it done.' She doesn't make eye contact and walks into the hairdressers' room. 'You will have it done later, Dorothy,' she says, returning.

It was clear from the heat of the day that this was the time of year when residents had more opportunity to get outside. Recently Dorothy had been out with Nancy for a picnic by a lake outside one of the pretty market towns nearby. Another local trip was also planned but Dorothy was undecided. And she only wanted to go with Nancy. In the main, Nancy took Dorothy's demands in her stride. Sometimes, though, Nancy's exasperation was palpable, and then she'd go on her break. These moments of ambivalence were often forgotten and Dorothy continued to recognise Nancy as her special 'Wendy'. Without Nancy in sight, Dorothy's anxiety mounted. No one else was good enough.

Nancy appears from the hairdresser's salon. Dorothy beckons Nancy over, 'Wendy, Wendy, Wendy.' She looks at Nancy who is close, and pulls her face down towards her, smiling. 'Look,' she says, proudly turning Nancy's head around to show me.

Nancy doesn't stay long and gets a bottle of water, takes a sip as if she is very thirsty. She walks over to the care assistant who stops hoovering. Nancy goes to the cupboard with the slings. The nurse returns. All three stand discussing slings; the nurse has one in her hand and is pulling it fully stretched out. Dorothy is watching all the while. 'Wendy, Wendy, Wendy,' she shouts, raising up her hand again to get their attention. Nobody turns.

Dorothy beckons the nurse over who is carrying the sling. She walks quickly towards Dorothy and starts adjusting her feet without speaking, placing both down flat on the footrests. Dorothy pushes the nurse off. 'Don't do that, don't do that, don't do that.'

Nancy reappears, asking Dorothy if perhaps they'll go to the garden centre later. Dorothy smiles, giving no formal response. Nancy drops the subject, as if it is just too hard. Nancy says that Dorothy's hair is messy. She walks into the hair salon and comes back with a comb. She shows it briefly to Dorothy and goes to the back of her head and starts combing.

'No, no, no,' says Dorothy, grimacing. 'That hurts, hurts, hurts.'

'But it's messy. Nearly done.'

'Don't do it, don't, don't.'

Nancy continues until it is combed through. 'It's better now,' says Nancy, smiling. Dorothy shakes her head, quietly bending her head down. Tears are forming in her eyes. This is a violation for Dorothy. She brings her head back up and looks ahead.

An activities co-ordinator walks past with a large board full of words. Dorothy beckons her over. She stops and explains that she has been playing word games. She invites Dorothy to join next time. 'You don't want that, you don't want that, you don't want that,' says Dorothy, looking at the big board.

The activities co-ordinator asks Dorothy if she wants to go out to the herb farm for a trip. Dorothy smiles, but doesn't seem to hear, so the subject is dropped. The activities co-ordinator goes.

A young male carer in his twenties comes along.

Dorothy makes a strange howling sound; he shrugs his shoulders. He stands at the nurses' station. Another female carer, clothes tightly fitting, comes along and also stands by the station. Nancy returns and stands there too. All mumbling, words blur.

'Wendy, Wendy, Wendy,' shouts Dorothy, looking over at them. 'No, no, no,' she says. No one responds. Dorothy begins to push her feet down on the ground, off her footrests. 'I want to get out, get out, get out,' she says. 'I want to go home.' She stops.

The hairdresser walks out of the salon. 'Hello,' she says, beaming. 'That's right, that's right, that's right,' says Dorothy, looking at her.

A lunch waiter pushes a trolley past. Moments later the chef, with his hat and black and white chequered trousers, walks past with several plates of food. He wheels them into the dining room.

The activities co-ordinator wheels a woman past Dorothy and asks her if she wants to look out of the window. 'There you are, there you are, there you are,' says Dorothy. The activities co-ordinator stops, leaves the resident in the middle of the corridor, at sea, and doubles back to say hello to Dorothy. 'Hello,' she says, holding out her hand to her. They hold hands momentarily. Dorothy smiles: touch, contact, essential.

Another carer wheels another woman through into the lounge. The young male carer follows and stands behind the women. He talks momentarily to her then begins to kick a red ball around behind them in the lounge, as if practising football on his own, a kid in an empty playground. Dorothy watches.

Nancy moves around the nurses' station, leaving her colleagues, and begins to drink from the bottle of water. She finishes it. It is now empty. 'Wendy, Wendy, Wendy,' says Dorothy, raising up her hand again. She points at the empty bottle of water and opens out her hands as if to play catch. Nancy throws the bottle and Dorothy catches it, startled. She throws it back to Nancy. The male carer comes in, leaving the red ball behind. Dorothy points to the bottle, 'That's what you were doing, doing, doing.'

'You want to hit me with it?' says the young male carer, pretending to be nervous.

'No,' corrects Nancy, 'she wants to throw it.'

Nancy and the young male carer and Dorothy form a three and do a bit of catching. 'Where is the ball?' asks Nancy. The male carer explains where it is. Nancy goes off to get it while Dorothy watches. Nancy returns with the ball and throws it to Dorothy, who frowns. She throws it back to Nancy then picks up her orange juice. Nancy is about to throw it. 'No more of that, of that, of that,' says Dorothy. 'I have a glass,' she says assertively, clearly. No repetition.

'Oh all right,' says Nancy, laughing. She comes close to Dorothy and the young male carer sits on Dorothy's armrests. Nancy perches herself on the table at the right hand side. The young man fiddles with Nancy's bun, affectionately, and then asks Dorothy who I am. She ignores him. She puts her orange juice down and takes up her two hands, and gently strokes Nancy's face. 'Aargh,' says Nancy. Dorothy smiles. They sit in silence for a moment and Nancy explains that she might take Dorothy out later. 'That would be nice, wouldn't it?' Perhaps Dorothy will go out after all.

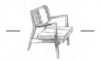

'You've got your toes,' she says, noticing my feet in flip flops.

'I have,' I say.

'That's right,' she smiles. Dorothy isn't repeating herself.

She tries to put her own burgundy-slippered foot back on the footrest, then gives up.

Nancy walks past with a bottle of water in her hands, with a different male carer. 'See you soon,' she says, going on her break. Dorothy doesn't seem phased.

The phone is going at the nurses' station, but the male carer doesn't answer it. He continues notetaking. Dorothy starts looking at some photos beyond the nurses' station: care workers on a works-do. 'That's lots of them,' she says.

'Johnny, Johnny, Johnny,' cries the woman next to Dorothy. The care assistant at the station looks up momentarily. 'It's all right, Evie.' He returns to his files.

The male carer leaves the nurses' station for a few minutes and goes into the cupboard behind the woman next to Dorothy. Dorothy watches him leaving and shakes her head.

'I don't know what I'm doing here. All on my own,' she says.

The male carer, who had gone to the lounge, appears and comes face to face with Dorothy, waving. Dorothy looks at him and, as he walks away, she sticks out her tongue. She laughs. 'That's what I do,' she says, 'that's what I do.'

Evie is still calling out. 'Johnny, Johnny, Johnny.' She makes a dreadful sound as if she is in pain. The other carer taps her gently on the head and tells her she is all right. She isn't. He walks straight past, back to his filing.

She briefly opens her eyes and fiddles around for the cup in front of her.

Dorothy puts her head onto the top of her hand and closes her eyes.

Nancy returns from her break and stands in front of Dorothy. Dorothy gradually opens her eyes. Nancy had not managed to get to work the week before because she had hurt her back. She is going to take it easy from now on. Since she has been away Dorothy is not bothered by her. It's true that Dorothy seems distant now. She hasn't called out 'Wendy' once.

Nancy says that she has got to go to another resident and walks around the corridor. Dorothy lets her go, no complaints. Dorothy does not follow her with her eyes but notices the tea man, who stops in front of her. He offers her a biscuit. She takes a chocolate one.

'That's right,' says Dorothy, 'that's right.' She takes a bite of her biscuit. When two crumbs fall she immediately wipes them from her jumper. Clean and tidy like Whittinghall.

The tea waiter moves onto Evie and offers her a biscuit and a tea. 'Johnny, Johnny, Johnny,' she calls. It's not biscuits that she wants.

Dorothy finishes chewing and notices one of the carers in front of her. He wants to know about the observations and whether the manager chose Dorothy as a subject. He moves around to Evie. He asks her to take her medication which is in a teacup, but she says it is too cold.

'Johnny, Johnny, Johnny,' she says. 'I want company.' He stops and bends down and holds both of her hands in his. This lasts a moment.

'She wants a cup of tea,' says Dorothy, trying to hear what they are saying. 'Cup of tea.'

The care worker offers to get her a warmer piece of toast.

'I am hungry,' she says.

'Do you want a biscuit?' he asks, 'or a nice warm piece of toast?'

She asks for toast. He stands up and as he goes past he stops in front of Dorothy and offers her a new cup of tea.

'Too hot,' she says, 'too hot, too hot.'

'Always repeating,' he says. 'She has dementia too.' That's his explanation for the repetition. Close it down.

She begins to put her head into her hands, closing her eyes again. 'Nice to see you, to see you,' she whispers, before falling into a deep sleep.

Nancy is sitting in one of the lounge chairs on her mobile phone, texting.

It seemed Nancy's week off was a sign that she had overstretched herself looking after Dorothy. She would take it easy now, take breaks, escape through her phone, relieve herself of the intensity of being Dorothy's 'Wendy'. The relationship had changed.

It was Bastille Day. In Whittinghall – in the middle of Middle England – the day went unmarked. Although it was reported that Dorothy could be aggressive, revolution and rebellion among the residents was not commonplace at Whittinghall. Most residents in Huntside unit kept themselves to themselves, behind closed bedroom doors. Those who appeared were often moving from A to B with the supervision of a member of the care team; residents who sat in corridors often slept, and very few walked around. The home was often quiet. Today was no different. In the absence of carers, Dorothy and Evie continued to sit on, without uprising.

The young nurse is in the nurses' station, looking over prescriptions. Dorothy is seated in her wheelchair next to the coffee table, and on the other side of the table to the left is Evie, seated in a red velvet chair.

Dorothy is sleeping. She has her head down towards her chest, but not touching, feet resting on the footstools of the wheelchair. She is breathing deeply. Nancy appears and immediately starts to explain that Dorothy is getting increasingly violent during personal care. You wonder whether this has to do with the bond between them, a bond that's breaking. Nancy says that it is very hard work. She is on the receiving end; everyone is now. Dorothy has her own allocated psychiatric worker, to help make things better. A professional has been brought in now.

Dorothy continues to sleep in the same position. The male cleaner is hoovering with a blue hoover that has a smiley face on it. It looks out of place in the sleepy corridor. Dorothy's one eye twitches momentarily, but she continues sleeping.

One of the male carers walks back into the corridor, gesturing that he might wake Dorothy, but it is decided to leave her be. Dorothy's feet are still, as is every part of her body, apart from the deep breathing, rising and falling. The nurse is still behind the station and the male carer is now searching for his drink, which looks like a smoothie, in his own bottle. Here carers take the time to refuel on the job. They use their own bottles, colourful and translucent, never the cups or glasses that belong to the home, to the residents.

'You are here, you are here,' Dorothy says on waking. She keeps her eyes locked on me for some time, as if she is coming to. She takes some time and picks up her left hand and smooths down the black cardigan she is wearing. She turns to her left and notices Evie, who is taking another bite of toast. 'What's she got there?' says Dorothy, pointing to the cup of tea and the water.

She looks down to her left and notices a glass of apple juice. She reaches over, picks it up, takes a drink. The nurse at the station stands up with the prescriptions in her hands. 'There she is, there she is,' says Dorothy, beckoning the nurse over. 'Hello,' she says, pushing her hand into the air and making her birdlike gesture with her fingertips. The nurse smiles and begins to walk past. 'Will you come, will you come?' says Dorothy out loud. The nurse walks backwards, slowly, and stops with Dorothy and asks her if she is alright.

'Yes I am,' says Dorothy. The nurse reaches out and holds Dorothy's hand. She stands like this for a minute then releases Dorothy's hand, and walks in through a door behind Evie. Feeling yourself existing in relation to another, we forget the meaning of such small acts.

The tea lady walks past but without the tea trolley. People and things are going missing.

Dorothy looks; pulls a face as if to say, 'What's she doing?' 'I don't know what I'm supposed to be doing. I don't know what I'm supposed to do.' The phone ringing endlessly, the tea lady without her trolley, a nurses' station without nurses, things are getting more confusing for someone already confused. Dorothy is pushing herself forward, saying that she can't see properly round there. How easy it would be to offer to walk Dorothy around the corner in her chair, to take her for a stroll and to satiate her curiosity, to ask the question and find the tea, the biscuits, the things she is used to right now at this time of day.

Evie is calling out. The male care worker appears. 'Help me, help me,' says Evie. He asks her what she wants. 'I need the toilet, the toilet,' she says. He asks her to stand up, 'One, two, three.' She finishes by saying, 'four, (fooooooour), five,'. She stands. Evie takes two steps and says she will have to sit down. She is struggling, sighing, calling out. 'Help me, Johnny, help me.' The carer pulls her zimmer-chair combo and asks if she wants to sit down. She does and thumps down on the seat. He begins to push her, but she complains. He stops and asks her if she wants to walk with him. 'Ooooh,' she says. A younger man with dementia walks in and begins talking to the male carer about his room. The male carer doesn't make eye contact with the man but starts following him to where he needs to go, leaving Evie in the chair in the middle of the corridor. Abandoned. She says nothing, her feet dangling from the chair.

'Don't like the look of that,' says Dorothy, noticing Evie's predicament. She shakes her head. The phone starts going again but no one answers.

'Can you ask me? Can you ask me?' cries out Dorothy, directing her questions to two members of staff deep in conversation at the nurses' station. No one hears her. She rests her head on her two forefingers on her left hand and stays there, head bent for some time. You wonder if it is always aching.

When no one hears or sees your rebellions, do you just give up?

Several weeks passed, summer holidays. Children out of school and care workers taking breaks meant that there had been some disruption. In the outside world there were changing contexts: uniforms were off and schoolbooks left in bags. Inside Whittinghall though, routines generally stayed on track and, though some familiar faces were absent, the day-to-day tasks and rhythms continued. However, there was one new development that was creating an unspoken anxiety in the home.

The young nurse is at the nurses' station, looking over a file. Dorothy is in her wheelchair in her usual position. Evie has gone. For now. This time a man is to the left and a woman with dark-black rimmed glasses in the chair to the right. Dorothy is sandwiched between two people who are sleeping.

The man has a piece of untouched toast in front of him, cut into four fingers, and an empty cup of tea. 'There you are,' she says, surprised that I have come again. She picks up her orange juice and raises it, still smiling. 'Get out,' she says, showing me the orange juice. Her facial expression and words don't necessarily marry up, but perhaps say something about ambivalence.

The nurse puts her head up and smiles too. She hasn't had her holiday yet but is looking forward to one.

Nancy is on a break. Another senior carer comes in and chats with the nurse about the new system. The nurse begins talking to her about the unit being short-staffed. Another carer comes along and stands where the male carer was a moment ago. A carer from the dementia unit next door arrives and begins talking to the nurse. There is some discussion about renegotiating shifts. The young nurse is explaining that two people are off sick. Another person is not able to come into work because they don't have a visa yet. She is overworked. On 7th and 8th September 2015, 130 care staff were targeted for overstaying their visas (28th September 2015, *Guardian*); of them, thirty-five Nigerian care workers will be detained. Many will have worked in the UK for over a decade and will be distraught about leaving behind older vulnerable people with whom they have forged close bonds; many of the older people will be wondering where those people who knew them so well have gone.

Nancy is standing opposite Dorothy, smiling at her. Dorothy points to her own arms. Nancy knows. She touches Dorothy's right arm, and asks her if she is cold. 'Yes, I am, cold, cold, cold.' Nancy says that she will get her a cardigan.

Nancy returns with the cardigan and tells Dorothy she has got something to make her warmer. 'Here you are, love,' she says. Dorothy looks. She holds out her arm and Nancy puts it on her arm, making sure it fits through the hole. She brings it round Dorothy's back but it is stuck on Dorothy's shoulders. 'She won't bend forward,' says Nancy. She struggles to put her right arm through the cardigan for a minute. Dorothy's arm looks a little awkwardly positioned, but she says nothing. The arm fits through finally. Nancy touches Dorothy's back, as if to prompt her to move forward. Dorothy bends far enough forward to allow Nancy to pull the cardigan down, flattening it down behind her back.

The woman from reception is asking the young nurse, who is visited by another young nurse, how to find out on the new system who has cleaned a certain resident's teeth. Dorothy is watching, eyes glued. 'I can see it,' she says. 'Can you?'

Nancy demonstrates where this kind of information can be kept on the system. She gets out her tablet device and shows the receptionist, who we suspect is a representative of the manager, Amy. The woman from reception goes on to explain that if she sees someone with hair all messed up she can now check whether the hair had been done in the first place. Nancy makes a joke about 'getting people into trouble'. These devices, we imagine, are a new form of surveillance. 'This is really what the new technology is there for,' says the receptionist. She has been asked by the manager to 'spot check'. She gives another example of an imagined woman without her imagined set of dentures in and someone saying they have cleaned the imagined set of teeth. Nancy reiterates her point about people getting into trouble. The receptionist laughs, 'Well, people could have forgotten, benefit of the doubt first.'

There are now four people at the nurses' station, discussing the new system.

The man next to Dorothy is still sleeping, but his body is plunging forwards ever so often. His forehead is nearly touching the table in front of him.

The young nurse has the new tablet device out and is talking about adding something to it. The young nurse who is sitting on the stool has hers out too. Both are looking at them and pressing different icons, as if they are playing Candy Crush. 'I have to do all the rotas; there is so much sickness, meds, the care plans. She could just do at least...' The young nurse feels that someone, we are not sure who, has let her down.

Nancy returns, looking at her tablet system, pressing the buttons. It pings when she has added something. Another nurse appears with the tablet attached to her belt and starts talking to the nurse behind the station. Nancy is moving her head from side to side and smiling, trying to make Dorothy laugh. Dorothy stares right at her, but gives away nothing. She is not playing the game.

A male carer appears. He has his tablet device out and is asking Nancy what he should put down. She explains that he needs to click the 'name' then 'wheelchair' and then 'activities'. The multitude of details from the morning condensed into a series of easy categories. He walks off studying the device, and you wonder whether the studying of people will take second place.

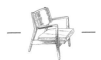

The activities co-ordinator hears the trolley come around, and explains to everyone that they are waiting for biscuits. Biscuits are like Huxley's delicious soma. Residents aren't talking to one another around the table, and it feels as though everyone is waiting for something to happen. An activity of flower arranging has been going on, and for once Daphne is part of it.

'Here he is,' says the activities co-ordinator. A man dressed as a waiter comes in. He parks up his trolley in the mini-kitchen area and picks up a tray of biscuits. He comes to Dorothy first, handing her a digestive. Immediately she takes a bite and gently chews the biscuit, sweeping any crumbs from her chest.

The waiter walks over to Dorothy with a new cup of tea, taking her old one away. She pushes the tea towards me and turns and smiles, 'Go on,' she says. This is a sign of friendship.

The activities co-ordinator finishes feeding the man in the wheelchair tiny crumbs of cake so that he does not choke. 'My darling,' she says and then puts her face towards him, almost touching foreheads. He looks at her, half smiling, half bemused. She walks away.

At times like these you wondered whether Dorothy could ever be herself at Whittinghall; or whether the man in the wheelchair felt at home enough just to cry out and shout, 'Give me the bloody cake.' Whatever the case, Dorothy seemed to have experienced yet another eviction – this time not from her country of origin, or her home, or even the more complete room of her mind. But the corridor. The movement – chosen or not – from the corridor to the lounge where the activities were taking place had made her feel homeless and she needed to return. Dorothy never mentioned her mother, but today she was summoning up her former role as a mother. Maybe those were the days when she had felt most at home.

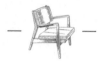

Amy, the manager, had been a shadowy figure, only ever seen that first day. Today, the final day, she reappears. For some weeks Nancy had also become a shadowy figure in Dorothy's life, but there had been a rapprochement: some warmth had been restored; repair following rupture.

Dorothy is seated in the corridor, opposite the nurses' station. She has her head bent and eyes closed, sleeping. The manager is resting her arms on the side of the nurses' station, talking to the lead nurse in the unit. She notices Dorothy, sleeping. 'Dorothy,' she calls to her. Dorothy slowly brings her head up and looks in the manager's direction, with barely a glint of recognition. She then turns to look at me, and smiles. I walk over to Dorothy and ask her how she is. 'I'm fine,' she says. 'How are you?'

Next to Dorothy is Evie again. She is calling out, 'Johnny, Johnny, Johnny.' A male carer goes towards her and the manager also walks to her. The carer pulls out Evie's chair-come-zimmer frame in front of her, asking her to stand. Evie is very shaky on her thin bruised legs, wobbling as she comes to a standing position, even with the help of the male carer. 'Johnny, Johnny,' she shouts. The manager is trying to explain something but as she does so laughter is leaking out of her. Evie turns and sits down on the chair part of the zimmer frame. 'No,' says the manager, 'Evie, this isn't a chair; this is your walking aid. Try to stand and you can walk to your room.' Evie looks puzzled. The seat that opens up as part of the zimmer frame is not a seat? The male carer is prompting Evie to walk, with his hand behind her back, firm but gentle. She begins to stand again. He and the manager help Evie to turn and to hold onto the handles of the equipment. 'You can walk now, Evie.' Slowly, Evie, with the male carer behind her, starts to move.

The manager returns to the nurses' station. Nancy walks into the corridor. 'Hello,' she says to Dorothy. Dorothy looks delighted to see her and puts her hand up into the air to wave. 'It's you, yes it is,' she says. 'It is me,' says Nancy, as if they are meeting after some time apart.

Nancy bends in close to Dorothy and smiles at her. Dorothy smiles back. 'What you doing?' asks Dorothy. 'I have got to do some work,' says Nancy. She walks over to the nurses' station and starts talking with the manager and the nurse behind the station. They seem to be discussing the new mobile phone devices; that one was already broken.

Dorothy shakes her head as she looks at them, and begins to close her eyes. Her proximity to the nurses' station was both comforting and isolating at the same time.

The manager turns around and notices Dorothy sleeping. 'Dorothy,' she punctures her sleep. 'You have a visitor.' Dorothy looks towards the manager. She looks at me and then looks in front of her, noticing a small glass of orange juice. She reaches down to try to pick it up but can't quite make it. Reaching for it on her behalf is the only thing to do. 'Thank you,' she says. She raises the glass to her lips and so very slowly tips the glass up. The orange juice moves closer towards her lips but very slowly. As the orange juice touches Dorothy's lips she almost sucks it in then swallows. She takes only a small sip before putting the glass back down on the table.

The manager is still at the nurses' station talking to the nurse about the broken mobile device. A male carer, who is going by with a trolley full of towels and flannels, stops in front of the station. He overhears the conversation. 'You broke my device, Dorothy,' he says and laughs. It is up to us to fill in the jigsaw.

The manager leaves.

The gentleman who has been in the corridor more recently is seated in his wheelchair, bent forward. His head is resting on the table in front of him and, though his eyes are closed, he is grumbling about something.

Dorothy is looking at her feet; one burgundy slipper is not quite in position on the footrest and she begins to get it into place. She moves it a few millimetres further up the footrest but it looks too hard. She gives up. She sits back in her chair. Then she sits very much further forward, and makes as if she is going to stand up. She sits back down.

The tea trolley comes and stops in front of Dorothy. She smiles as the tea waiter hands her a digestive. She immediately brings it to her mouth and takes a small bite. A couple of crumbs fall down her top and she sweeps them off with her right hand. No mess, Dorothy, no mess. Dorothy begins to fall asleep as if she knows my time is up and the visits are ending, for ever. She is taking control of this ending like she's taken control of most of the minor rejections she has experienced in these last few weeks.

TIME

Articulating unbecoming through breathlessness,
Shuffled feet and heads bent down at floors cleaned
Tirelessly by proud people tired by cuts.
Swallowed up by velvet chairs and foreheads leaning
Into cold toast on tables with wheels.
Noises in the background, antiques in attics
Discovered by loud voices and celebration
While we sit on, blankets covering legs with muscle waste.
'I need a wee,' we hear you but we cannot help.
Someone in uniform, gloves on
And ready. After doing one, two, three, four already.
Trolleys feeding numbers with false teeth
And changing tastes. No wine now.
Cabbages, cabbages, cabbages
But we are not that. Articulating our unbecoming
We say, 'Take a seat with us and share
The silence that welcomes us in.'
Dog howls and rushes through
In chase of pigeons or slippered feet.
A balloon is batted past our heads and kicked
By someone younger. This is play
Still for us in chairs.
'What is this life, if full of care,'
She mumbles, 'We have no time to stand and stare.'
'No, quite right,' he laughs, 'Sit down.'

3 February 2015

During the months that I visited Winston Grove and Whittinghall, I was regularly taken up with the need to put some echoes of the work into poetry form. Being compelled to write like this was instinctual. It was a response to being stirred up by the experience of being with the people in these homes, reliving the experience through the material. Individual residents came to mind, as did members of staff: the smells, sounds, bodily gestures, as well as stories of past and present. The poetry attempted to make sense of what I had witnessed, creating a patchwork of memories, stringing events together, reconstructing and reconnecting time and space, even if in reality they didn't unfold like that.

I say this because what follows is the attempt to produce something more orderly, a thematic narrative, coherent and analytical. To articulate what was going on organisationally through individual and collective minds is a difficult task; the more you feel you begin to know, the more questions arise, the more the knowing feels out of reach. It was this not-knowing that drove me to verbalise the experience poetically. It spoke to the muddle, confusion and non-linearity of being in care homes for people with dementia. That is not to say that it was impossible to isolate certain qualities of care, but rather that extrapolating clear themes does not do full justice to 'being there' and 'speaking with' because being there and speaking with also allowed me to see where paradoxes and contradictions existed, where omissions occurred, and why it was so hard to make claims to truths.

Being with Daphne at Winston Grove, and Dorothy and Nancy at Whittinghall, meant sitting and walking, experiencing with them. Although I was seeing their lives and relationships through my own eyes, there were times when the full weight of pain or joy that they encountered felt as if it had penetrated my own psychic skin. These were moments when my identification with either Daphne or Dorothy allowed me momentarily to forget my own identity as a younger person, with children, in a relatively healthy body, and imagine myself in their shoes.

Speaking with staff and residents more formally did not lend itself to the same depth of identification – words perhaps, and the taking up of the 'researcher' role, gave me less scope for 'self-fragilising' (Ettinger, 2006). The reliance on language, a system that interprets and abstracts feeling and lived experience, meant that I too felt more distant.

Yet time with Dorothy and Daphne, just sitting and walking, led to discoveries which were often made through an attunement to moods, flows, sound, rhythmical movement – through the unspoken, pre-symbolic. In conversation, an increased focus on words, and the cognitive, sometimes led to an engagement of my thinking mind more than my feeling one.

That said, there were stand-out incidences, when I spoke with people, where feelings were powerfully communicated: Sue, at eighty, trying to return to Wales on the bus to get to school; Ellen struggling to match up her shoes, claiming my foot as her own; Diane likening care work to the relentless brutality of the Holocaust and other forms of racism, and Sophia trying to come to terms with death. These conversations slowed me down, opened me out to the speakers' lives. But relationships are funny things and one major component of them is time. I wondered how much more I would have learned if there had been more time.

Since words are at the basis of talking, the semantic losses of older people showed up time and time again, occasionally a conversation became more like a puzzle. During and afterwards, I felt I had to fill in gaps to create more recognisable meaning. How hard it must be to live with, or work with, the puzzle and its ill-fitting pieces. The process reminded me of the meaning-making that may go on between an infant, 'before words', and a mother. In a dementia care context, the maternal figure – if we are to call it that – helps to hold and to define meaning when someone is communicating 'after words'. This involves being attuned enough to another human being to be able to express what that 'inexpressible' thing might be.

What some carers try to do, with the voices of the people with dementia, is to create a coherent narrative where sometimes such a narrative is elusive. This involves a 'holding' together of strands. We might be reminded of Winnicott (1960) and 'going-on-being'; how a relatively continuous sense of self is central to our lives; how, with dementia, meaning might escape us and we may need help to reconstruct it. It was a great privilege to have these conversations with residents and staff, and to find a shape, together, to the organisations they worked and lived in, and which simultaneously inhabited them.

The daily grind of the work was thoughtfully spoken about: the pressures; the ideals; the austere regimes. For some, words seemed to allow them to mask some of the hardships of care work. Nancy, who at times struggled with Dorothy, resisted thinking about her ambivalence. One or two gave glossy interviews, containing 'advertising speak' of the kind we might find in marketing brochures for care homes.

Staff, as they talked, seemed more self-conscious, processed, whereas material from the observations involved more leaks and slippages. Movements into the unconscious were present in discussions through involuntarily bodily movements, coughing, laughing, and staff members sometimes used powerful images to convey ideas about the care homes.

Residents with dementia seemed less defended. Protective defences, perhaps assumed to be part of 'sane' adult subjectivity (Phillips, 2005, p. 69), seemed to be diminishing. Conversations were often raw, capturing emotional realities rather than factual ones. This mirrored my experience of being in the homes, particularly when residents searched for mothers on difficult days.

TICK-TOCK

Time, as the reader will have seen, was ever-present at Whittinghall. Dorothy, herself, was seated opposite a clock. The long hand of the clock felt as if it were barely moving each week. This focus on time related to the overall, sometimes paralysing, sense of waiting at Whittinghall. Ironically, the staff team never seemed pressed for time. Time was heavy and available, yet the availability of time was not necessarily used in service of the residents.

In Winston Grove, there was little evidence of staff breaks. Staff spoke about the lack of time, and seemed to be permanently busy doing one thing or another. They needed more time for dressing, more time for playing and feeding, time for training and reflection.

At both sites, the residents tended to exist out of linear clock-time, revisiting earlier periods of their own history. Residents, when they spoke, often tried to bridge the gap between the present and the past. The future was never thought about.

In talking with staff, a clear link was made between the conceptualisation of time-as-brutalising and the sense of an occupational death as a symptom of austerity measures; and for the residents there was a need to access time to do some gentle mourning in the presence of a responsive other.

Competing notions of time often caused organisational tensions. This was particularly evident when residents' needs, many immediate, were at odds with the home's routines, time-tabled according to linear clock-time. In Winston Grove, there was a greater rebellion against time constraints. Sometimes carers, particularly in Daphne's unit, seemed to slow it down deliberately. This happened a few times during lunchtime. At Whittinghall, time was generally more available, owing partially to the greater number of staff on shift. Staff took more breaks from the work, and were often seen drinking from their own bottles as if refuelling. This availability of time, yearned for at Winston Grove, did not mean that staff at Whittinghall made more contact with residents. On the contrary, the staff took the opportunity to congregate together around the nurses' station, as peers.

At Winston Grove, references to time and its significance in and for care work were frequent. A common association was made between good care and time spent with residents or time given to staff. Many carers talked longingly about 'one-to-one' time; a short-hand for a form of rewarding relating where both parties could exchange personal details. These almost sacred encounters were considered scarce and in counterpoint to the general busyness of care work and its associated tasks. At Winston Grove, carers were saddened by the reality that time was becoming increasingly stretched: at least one floating shift (covering breakfast) had been cut, leading to what they described as 'conveyor-belt care'. At Whittinghall, time was not mentioned.

The experience of linear time was shaky for all residents. The fact that, at Whittinghall, the staff team had placed a 'day of the week' sign up for Dorothy demonstrated how precarious temporal markers were. People with dementia seemed to exist in the moment without an external temporal frame; time was internally defined and as a result many retreated to times that had long since passed.

Care staff's relation to time

BRIDGET

Bridget, a long-standing member of staff, doubles up as a cleaner and she also assists at mealtimes. She is a vocal woman, often prompting carers to respond to residents. She has done her breakfast shift and wants to talk in the activities room, a colourful space in the home, at the end of a corridor. There are paintings on the walls. This is where the activities co-ordinator, Gemma, sometimes runs craft and ball groups. Bridget laughs a lot.

Bridget imagines herself as holding a privileged position within the organisation, as the mealtime work affords her a slower pace, the chance to be with the residents. Bridget talks a lot about her perceived place in the organisation, and how it relates to time.

'It's nice, here. Residents are nice. A lot of the staff are nice. Um, I do enjoy it. There are different aspects to my work that I do.' In the room, a resident stands behind her, mumbling something. He moves from one foot to the other. Bridget smiles, noticing him standing behind her. He then leaves. 'So I spend a lot of time with the residents in the morning and then during the day I'm just doing my work. I sit, chat, laugh, joke and we sing sometimes.' Bridget can't help but break into laughter but it is unclear why. 'It depends how somebody's feeling and… so this is all happening while we're doing breakfast.' She laughs again, perhaps at multiple demands on her time, all the different types of nurturing expected of her.

Bridget is clear that all the staff need more time, and that one-to-one time with residents is a privilege. '… They don't get it during the day 'cos obviously there's lots going on during the day and it can get overlooked. Yeah, I can get someone to do something that you can't [laughs]. 'Cos I have more time 'cos obviously carers are busy… they're doing the basics whereas I don't have to do the basics.' She defines herself quite apart from the carers.

'Personal care, I don't do any of that,' she says. 'I would call a carer to come and do that… And I don't do medication, anything like that, that a resident is going to associate with a carer. I have the nice bit. I'm going to give you something to eat and we're going to have a laugh and a joke whereas a carer doesn't have that time 'cos they've got eight to ten residents on their unit that they need to be giving personal care to…'

In the background one of the home's dogs is in a cage in the room, squealing. It becomes hard to concentrate but Bridget carries on explaining that she has the fun bits of the work; her role is different. She has this expanse of time which affords her all sorts of entry points into the relational. Bridget explains that 'although some people may not be able to string a whole sentence together, if you listen carefully and you've got one-to-one with somebody who can't string a sentence together you can make sense of what it is they're trying to say so you can work out what it is they want and you get that smile at the end of it rather than an aaargh.' Bridget is enacting some kind of roaring. She's powerful right now. 'That's why I think it's important if you can spend time with residents… I think it's great even if they don't make sense but neither do we at times.' She has got a point. In fact, among the brouhaha of the dog squealing and another *resident coming in, Bridget imparts some gems. 'Oh, it's knowing the little things… and I know little things because I've seen somebody kick off and it's like ooh, now, why did that happen? And I can take time to retrace why… I might have said something wrong or I've said "yes" when they're trying to tell me "no" so you think, "oh fine, that means no then" …you pick up on how they're trying to tell you.'*

(Winston Grove)

The organisation-in-the-mind (Armstrong, 2005) for Bridget is one that is hurried, in which carers find minimal time to spend with the residents, yet fun and understanding is available, at least in her role. The one-to-one possible at breakfast gives Bridget the opportunity to engage in play, laughter, singing with residents. Time is seen as a way into connection.

Despite her formal working role as a cleaner, Bridget conveys a sense of authority. Her formal role might have been associated with a lack of education, with a lowly position in the organisational hierarchy, but Bridget's sense of agency was impossible to miss. She makes claims to know the residents and to be able to work with them in a way that others could not (she knows more than 'you'). She asserts her position yet, perhaps beneath the voice of authority, she is regretful that she is a cleaner. She seems to have more to offer. Her nervous laughter possibly communicated something about the riskiness involved in stepping out of role.

It seemed that her sense of authority related to her ability to claim time within the organisation, and to know the residents well. The time which was available to Bridget also linked with her desire to be considered superior to carers. Bridget wanted others to see in her a breadth of capacities which weren't commonly associated with cleaning, and we might wonder how issues of class and race feature in her thinking. It was as if she could not bear the possible powerlessness that a housekeeper's position might have implied in terms of the hierarchical dimensions of Winston Grove. To think of Armstrong (2005), Bridget's organisation-in-the-mind was populated with categories of hierarchy that were seemingly crafted by local government, and which led to splits and the punctuation of interpersonal space around both role and task, in her case.

That said, people conducting domestic duties in care homes, nursing homes, palliative care environments, are often able to make genuine, and important, contact with 'patients' when nurses or carers are busy with other tasks.

At Winston Grove, the spontaneity, the play that Bridget alludes to was part of the culture of the home. For Bridget, relating like this, supported by time, facilitated knowing and discovering. She herself makes the association between meaning-making and time. The home is a place in which coherence is sometimes out of reach, where residents are not able to string sentences together. Bridget believes she contributes to meaning-making through attending to, and accepting, the unlinked communications from residents in play.

This access to time seemed to offer her, and staff like her, a protected space within the organisation. This was linked to a belief that those with time at their disposal could achieve greater connection through play, the social, than those hurriedly on-task. Of course, Bridget made an important case for human contact in a care environment, and it did seem a reality that she was not as rushed as the carers. Nonetheless, Bridget seemed to align herself with workers like Gemma.

Gemma was the activities co-ordinator at Winston Grove, another member of staff who presented herself as someone able to create connections, in contrast to the rushed care staff. There were some overlaps with Bridget's material, an agreement that time offered a better quality of relating. Gemma, however, had many qualifications and, despite her formal education, she seemed less confident in her role within the organisation than Bridget did.

GEMMA

Gemma likened herself to a 'nanny and granddad' because she had the time to have 'fun' with the residents. Gemma is relatively young. She has worked in home care, nursing care, and residential care since completing her studies. She does not often do the 'basics'. She takes residents on local trips to the shops, cafes, and parks. She has just finished a game of bingo with a group of residents.

Gemma stops our conversation midway fearing that she is not responding 'right'. Was Gemma concerned that I would be critical of her explanations, fearful that her job didn't involve enough of the 'real work'?

Gemma talks about a successful example of her work, taking time to get to know a resident in preparation for a celebration. In counterpoint, she presents a picture of heavy daily care work.

Gemma is smiling. 'So… we did some research with her daughter… we got the family involved… a lady who once lived in China… really enjoyed that day and her family actually came and enjoyed it with her. Joined in which was nice... it gave us activities and like arts and crafts... we made a Chinese dragon. We looked into how... what Chinese dragons look like and how they were decorated, and the colours... painted dragons and put them up. It was quite good. So all the residents got involved in various different ways... And then people were experiencing... that they may not have experienced before... and because it had food involved it went down very well.' She smiles and breaks into laughter. 'It was, like, something for, um, all the senses.'

A male resident, fond of Gemma, walks in, stands behind her coughing. He leaves when he notices that she is doing something.

Gemma looks as though she wants to say more, but can't quite bring herself to do so. Then... 'And some people just don't realise that... They think, Oh I've done my job... they're dressed, fed, watered ... we'll just leave them in front of the TV. [Brief pause.] What kind of a life is that really? They may as well... just existing.'

Gemma looks pensive, and then speaks again, countering her earlier critical remarks. 'I think it is back-breaking work... not enough carers, even in a care home that's fully staffed... I don't think there's never enough... People tend to run around and pass people in the corridors, say hi as they're going past... as a carer they always seem, it's that side of them... Oh they've not got up, they're not dressed and they've not had their breakfast. Their concentration is doing that side of it. I think they need to have more concentration... with people... stimulating them, talking to them, making them feel special, making them feel like they're wanted... they feel they have hardly any time to get things done.'

She is thinking about care workers and trying to work out what is going on. This moment's conversation gives her space for reflection. She sees the routinisation of care, she understands the social context this is happening in. 'Yeah, because in a care home you only have so many staff that are allocated to so many residents and people try to [muffled word]... and cutting costs and things like that... um, where am I going with this now?... it gets a bit more regimented so you have lunch at one o'clock. Now you don't have to have lunch at one o'clock but people make them try to have their lunch at one o'clock 'cos it makes it easier. And 'cos there is a lot... there are a lot of people in this home... so forty-three people and you've got two carers per unit, which is what two, four, six, seven, eight carers and you've got your domestic staff on top. It's pushing it... because there are high levels of needs, you know. A lot of people aren't able to... put on their own clothes and give themselves a wash.'

This is the reality of care, the people at Winston Grove are often extremely dependent; they need time. Gemma knows this. *'...we've got people who are hoist dependent... completely dependent on you to.... you know... carers are running round, trying to tidy their bedrooms as they go... make sure they've eaten, make sure they've had a drink, they've had their medication.'* She pauses. *'It's hard. They need someone who can just be around to... a member of staff available so they can get that person up with no rush. So that time's not rushed...'*

(Winston Grove)

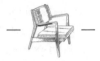

Time is associated with pleasure, and activity. In Gemma's mind, she is involved in a form of relating that is relatively free from conflict. On one level, Gemma expresses real empathy with busy carers. She talks of the back-breaking work. They are positioned as task-driven and time-impoverished; up against the clock. On another level, she is quietly critical of carers, imagining them forcing time on residents for their own convenience. Again we see an organisation-in-the-mind imbued with splitting and division – a psychic and relational process organised by the structuring of tasks by time.

These distinctions were sometimes observable on visits, but there were many examples that challenged the neat split that Gemma perceived. During one exercise activity, Gemma herself was outpacing the residents, jokingly calling them 'wet lettuce(s)' for their slow movement.

Contrary to Gemma and Bridget's representation of carers, there was a great deal of evidence of carers slowing down time to accommodate the needs of residents, where there was a careful pacing that mirrored residents' experiences. One poignant moment was when Bridget the housekeeper, the deputy manager Lynn, and a care worker, Erica, all stopped to make time for an encounter with Daphne that, though brief, was meaningful, where Daphne's greeting 'Hey Ho the Barley Mow,' acted as a catalyst for connection. As she took leave she expressed her gratitude with 'Thank you. Every loves.'

For Gemma time is understandably written into the kind of practice that allows residents to be treated well. Gemma talked about working in home care where she stretched time, sacrificing her own time, fighting quietly against service-provider timetabling. Choosing time becomes an ethical dilemma, one that can lead to worker exploitation. Other carers at Winston Grove talked about their mini-revolutions against time constraints. This ethical stance means that carers feel they are doing the right thing for residents, but organisationally they might be doing the wrong thing.

At the end of our talk, Gemma takes me aside to tell me how she would love to be in closer communication with her work colleagues. Gemma worries about being alienated and having to pull the psychosocial weight of the organisation. She did have a generative role within Winston Grove and sometimes active engagement with residents got located in her. However, carers also reported having meaningful encounters with residents, yet they approached intimacy in different ways. In actuality, Gemma was rarely alone, running the activities groups.

It is interesting to note that conversations with Gemma and Bridget were the longest out of all the members of staff. This seemed to indicate that carers were generally more hard-pressed than Gemma and Bridget were, and that the care workers did not always have time for slowed-down human interaction. However, the distinction (in terms of having time to relate) between their roles and the carers' was over-drawn.

There was one carer, Celia, who stood out, giving the longest interview of all carers. She was also the longest-serving member of staff at Winston Grove.

CELIA

The activities room was being used for staff training. Celia takes a chair in a sparse, cold room we have been provided with, and I sit on the edge of a chair to speak to her. A power dynamic already in play?

Celia takes pride in her work. She believes the work has to be done with great care. Although she had seen many changes in the home, appearing exasperated by many of them, her attitude to her work and to the residents was committed.

Celia is serious, speaking with conviction, with force. 'You give him a drink and he will calm down because he doesn't say, "Oh I'm hungry, I want something to eat", but he is like the same person. When I went to the new unit, to this one, all the handover was, "Didn't eat his lunch,* didn't eat" so I was under the thing of observing this situation then I observe, ok this man is coming down at 11am, washed and dressed, because of his meds he tends to sleep late and I'm not one for waking people up because what's the point of waking them up because they get all agitated. Let them sleep, give them whatever medication and then eventually get them up. This person comes down at 11am and that's where I talk about this hotel-model care, everything is done in this block of time. Hotel-model, that's what I call it. Or what happens in the hospital. Personal-centred care is not based on this. I observed him at 11 o'clock and then comes dinner at one and you sit him and give him his dinner, and he's not eating his dinner and they hand over, "Such and such didn't eat." Well, eleven, twelve, one, would you go and eat?' Celia looks astonished. 'After having had breakfast at eleven? Go having a big dinner, it's common sense. Stagger it.'

She goes on to explain the effects of having shifts cut, of being under greater pressure than before. 'Staff. That's the issue. It's the staff... in this unit... don't have like before a domestic that would help with the breakfast. I get in in the morning, we set up the tables, you get everything ready, porridge, then before you could go off. So for me one is up and one remains in the event of anything, one goes up to the residents, up, and one has to be down.' She is making a treatise on poor care, on care that concerns her, on care that cheats her and those she looks after. 'I don't mind that to a point, you know if you're not certain just ask to ... You know it's just you find yourself going and going and going all the time. Aaahhaaaaaahaaa [as if in pain]. It has its challenges, challenges in its own way. But what we need is continuity of staff and I think maybe it's all to do with them at the top and their finances, but make us work on a lesser staff ratio and don't expect the same because something is going to fall short. And if you are going to be on people's cases people won't be doing things the way it should be done. And um I don't know about conveyer-belt care, I know about person-centred care and that's what I'm going to do because I like to treat people the way I want to or would like to be treated if I cannot do things for myself any more. You know, so... I can't do it differently. If I go into help someone it has to be properly done. I don't do shortcuts.' Human beings cannot be treated as parts. 'So when somebody going to be taking ten and I'm taking fifteen, twenty because I'm allowing you, I'm showing you which one would you like to wear today? I'm not choosing that for you... And these things take time... Not you just rushing them. Let her do

what she wants, wash her five minutes, let her get on with it, maybe that's
how long she took to wash there. I cannot change because oh you want
this done in this time when the person wants this time. No I can't do it.'

(Winston Grove)

Celia points out that one of the reasons that there are more time pressures on her and other permanent staff is because a floating domestic shift has been removed. Getting the residents ready in the mornings feels like a production line (which she calls 'hotel-model' care – everything done in designated 'block[s] of time'). In order to provide the person-centred care (synonymous with empathy, attunement) in the way she would like, she makes the decision to resist hurrying the residents. There is a painful recognition that the practice of care is being distorted by economising, and, relatedly, increased demands on workers' time.

Celia has a sense of her practice being driven by an ethical imperative, which involves working at residents' pace and knowing them. This sits in tension with what she sees as the current demands on care workers, and 'splits' from the temporary workers.

Winston Grove had faced staffing issues; this was undeniable. Celia suggested that the number of temporary workers in the home affected the consistency of care provided. It also meant, for her, that the effort and time that permanent carers had spent getting to know the residents was undervalued organisationally, as if temporary workers could do the care in the same way, without the intimate knowledge of the residents' experiences. Perhaps the reader remembers the temporary carer unaware of and apparently unconcerned about Suki's needs to be toileted. How excruciating that had been for her.

Celia's relationship with time gives her a unique platform among the carers. She has worked in the home for over twenty years, experiencing many changes around care policy and practice. For Celia, working in older people's care had become increasingly difficult, in the face of resource cuts, more paperwork, and frequent changes of staff. Having survived the changes, her voice is strong and knowing. Her time in the home offered her a different sort of expertise to other carers I spoke with; I noticed myself hanging at times on her every word, as if she could tell me all about good and bad care.

There is a divide between the good old days, where work was perhaps more rewarding, and the present, a rushed, corner-cutting version of care. Celia's account no doubt had a rational, objective basis because she, like others, had witnessed funding cuts, poorer care, and a move from person-centred to more regulated forms of practice. Other distinctions were powerfully drawn, between temporary and permanent workers, hotel-model care and person-centred care. Yet the splitting, evident in her words, was also in some ways a retreat from thinking about the sadnesses that Celia might have been experiencing in terms of her own personal loss, having once had a valued occupational role. Her anger about the situation – as seen in these divisions into good and bad workers, types of care – nonetheless seemed to be an important position to hold on to. By feeling justified in her position, she was able to stage a daily protest against the time pressures she believed were eroding good care.

There were many other examples of splitting at Winston Grove. As well as splits between staff who 'have time' and those who 'do the basics', there were splits among residents as if some had a sense of the organisation as benign, and others a sense of it as being bad. (For instance, there was Ann who raged against the 'kids'' activities during a painting group and Daphne who wanted to express some gratitude for it.) It was possible that these tensions were symptomatic at times of a pervasive organisational paranoid-schizoid functioning (Klein, 1952).

Celia had the confidence to buck what she saw as the current system – hotel-model care wrapped up as person-centred care – in which carers were under pressure to 'do' people in ten minutes. Cutting time was related to the wider austerity agenda. Celia represented a quality of worker delinquency/rebellion that seemed part of the home. This was something of which workers and the manager seemed proud; equally, they consciously associated this stance as having an ethical underpinning. It was about making human lives better.

Celia's longevity in the home seemed to give her a robust sense of identity as a carer; she inhabited the role with self-possession as if she would not be beaten. Time was linked to wisdom, to identity.

Celia's voice was politicised. At a later stage she says, 'You cannot rush care; you cannot compromise care.' Celia implied that good care involved engagement, which was either restricted or supported by the availability of time and funds. When time is short, she argued, the quality of relating between carers and people with dementia is compromised, leaving both parties dissatisfied. It was black and white: good care seemingly couldn't be efficient and kind simultaneously.

Let me introduce you to another long-term carer, Diane, who reflects upon dementia care in the context of the wider political scene, regretful as she is about the way care is organised in austere times. She makes associations between the economic situation and the development of conveyor-belt care, which is personally burdensome, leaving her feeling unacknowledged in her work. The considerable time pressures are experienced as annihilating, a factor in a sort of occupational death.

DIANE

Diane has worked at Winston Grove as a carer for several years. At work, she moves slowly, unhurried, sometimes for her own benefit and sometimes for the residents. Diane has arranged cover after her morning shift, using her free-time to speak with me. Gemma is running a group activity so we sit in the activities room. Diane wants to speak, though she is conscious, apprehensive about the picture of Winston Grove she paints.

Her words roll out thoughtfully, seriously, yet she barely stops. 'You've got to understand the hierarchy and how it can affect you. Um. I enjoy working with people. I enjoy working with the elderly but it's a trend at the moment in the current economic crisis that they expect you to get somebody up out of bed, twenty minutes to half an hour, and washed and dressed and down to the breakfast table. I can't always do that.' Diane is re-imagining her shifts, the rushed mornings, the inconceivable speed at which carers are expected to work, how this jars with the pace of the older people in her care.

'What I will do, I will go to one. This person might tell me to pee off, not getting up now. I might be able to persuade them to have a biscuit and their medication, go to the next one. Next one might be the same. I have days when I go to two, three, four of them then I go back to the first, second, third one. They might be more approachable, put them on the commode, give them a cup of tea. Make them comfortable, go and do that with the next one. Then you might have someone who you can't put on the commode and you have to wash them on the bed. The bed might not be appropriate, it might be a back-breaker. You have to wash them, dry them, clean them, look after them, sort them all out, make them comfortable. Get them in a wheelchair, get them downstairs. You're expected to do your quota. Many a time I've been pulled up on it, but I don't take it personally.

Because it's not all about conveyer-belt care. It's about a quality of life that person has; it's about making it as pleasant and nice as possible for that person. It's about them; it's their time. So this is the problem that I have. Many a times I've been called into the office and given a bollocking. You can explain to them but they don't care. They're not interested. You've got to get a person down, twenty minutes to half an hour. What do you mean, you spent fifteen minutes and in that time you could only make someone a cup of tea and give them their medication, if they were willing to have? If they were not willing to have their medication, so what, I'll give it to them later. It's their time.' There is so much to think about, so much to do. It is hard to listen to Diane without considering the pressure she and others are under. Yet she doesn't pity herself; this seems to be the world of work for dementia carers each day.

'We're all in the same boat. You get some girls, whether they want to or they don't want to, washed, dressed, and brought downstairs. It doesn't matter if they can't wash them properly; it doesn't matter if they can't cream their skin properly. For me these people are very vulnerable; if I look after them and if I look after them well they'll last a bit longer and have a good life.' Diane refuses to speed up. She digs her heels in.

'But you get some of these super super people, fast, too fast, inflict their way regardless of how that person feels. You're getting up now, come on. Then they'll come and say "Di, I'm not like you, I got six up this morning and you only managed four." And I think, "shit, only managed four". Didn't hurt anybody, didn't bully anybody, didn't ride roughshod over anybody's needs... Treated them the same as I would treat my own mum or my own dad. They tell me to piss off or I'm not coming back to this hotel. Would you like a cup of tea? Cup of tea don't solve everything, huh, but I try anyway, try to make it as nice as possible.' She sounds angry. This is more complex work than making and serving teas: she knows that, as others do. But is this understood, the nuances of care, of good care?

'But you constantly feel of no value, constantly feel as though you are going against the grain. But for me these are human beings. When I get to ninety-four and I don't want to get out of bed, I won't get out of bed.'

(Winston Grove)

Diane points out that time belongs to the residents; carers should be sensitive to their pace. This bears striking similarities with mothering – the extra time it takes a toddler to sit in a car seat when he or she wants to do it themselves; the time it takes a small child to use a spoon at mealtimes... Who takes ownership of time, and the sequencing of daily life?

In the way she talks, without pause, Diane conveys something about the non-stop nature of the work, hurried, factory-like. The content of what Diane said contrasting with the way in which she speaks demonstrates powerfully how the treatment of time is divided: organisationally, there is a requirement, explicit or implicit, for speed; but for residents (and staff) this approach doesn't work.

The reader might remember Diane from Winston Grove, slowly offering up food to Gaynor, who had had a recent stroke. Gaynor recovered very well, which we might assume was testament to the time taken to care for her, as Diane notes above.

By holding time rather than speeding it up, we might notice that a greater amount of human agency can be encountered in the person with dementia. Diane firmly situates herself among the carers who revolt against time pressures, a troublesome individual (Symington, 2003) who has a rivalrous relationship with the 'super super people'. There were undoubtedly real differences between staff who prioritised human contact and those who were more instrumental, or compliant, in relation to management procedures. These differences had a footing in reality. However, the extent to which Celia and Diane seemed to conceive of the differences as entrenched and immovable also suggests a degree of splitting. This split meant they were able to deny their own task-focusedbehaviours, locating it fully in others. The situation was more complex than this. For instance, at Winston Grove almost everyone spoke fondly, in detail, about individual residents in their care, suggesting that relationships were important to workers across the board.

Diane also expresses a real capacity for empathy. She puts herself in the shoes of someone at ninety-four, who doesn't want to get out of bed. People of all ages do not always wish to fit into routine temporal structures and are entitled to say 'No'. Diane, in turn, is saying 'No' to those in the 'hierarchy'. Curiously, Diane encounters herself as both victimised and agential. She sees the residents in this way. Time is central to the argument: it can either become a persecutory object or a helpful one.

Diane's remarks about being in trouble with the manager fits with the idea that time can be used against care workers, as a way of judging their performance. She feels penalised by these judgements, linking in her mind the 'bollocking' with abuse. Diane suggests indirectly that time needs to be available, particularly in difficult, emotionally intense, situations. She references concentration camps and remembers racist notices posted on shopfronts. It is possible that Diane is capturing something that could not be thought or spoken about within the organisation.

'You know you only got four people up this morning and what do you think you were doing? Some of them have got dementia, some of them have got different mental problems. Some of them have different psychoses. Sometimes I might go into one resident, "You black bastard, you killed my mother, you killed my father, you killed the children I could have had. Don't touch me." And you start and calm them down and try and give them a cup of tea. But because of the way they feel you don't know if they might have had someone in a concentration camp, you don't know what the problem is. I'll take them out of their bedroom, take them to the dining room, ask the housekeeper, give them a cup of tea for their breakfast, please. And once she's calmed down I will try again or I'll get another carer and say if you get her washed and dressed for me I'll do one of yours.'

It is very noisy in the room; a carer and an elderly gentleman have come in. The dog is trying to get out of its cage, jumping up and down.

Diane is adamant. 'I am not going to do anything that makes me feel uncomfortable and make someone feel like shit so I can say, "hang on, I can score a brownie point". So, I don't know if I am the right person to be speaking to.' She tells me what it's like to be called a "black bastard" by people she is trying to look after.

'Well yeah I don't know what that's all about. But I know I didn't do it, whatever crime has been done. But I grew up back then, and I remember notices being up, not going in to shops. She's a bit older than me [Diane is talking about a particular resident] and it's possible she has had family that have been in the worst situations. Sometimes it's her worst nightmare and she worries about everything. Sometimes this lady can be sitting down eating her dinner and she says she's not eating, and she says, "What is this? I'm surrounded by blackies." And so I say to the activities co-ordinator, "Please sit down with her, chat to her, talk with her, have a dinner with." It's not my place to give her her dinner, chat to her, make her feel good. We've all got something in our cupboards that frightens us and it's a very lonely sad place to be but when I speak with my manager she says, "Well

next time it happens go and get one of the managers or the seniors to come
and witness it," but where you gonna find them? If there's a carer I'll say
"you hang on you're a white one, I'll relieve you," but we can't do our jobs.'
Perhaps none of us imagine that care work could be this intolerable at
times. Diane sounds frightened of being accused.

'Because if anybody comes in they might think you're abusing her,
doing something you shouldn't be doing, so there might be a problem with
safeguarding. I don't expect the manager to understand or even give me
any support. So I have to cover my own arse and protect myself.' Diane
makes an implicit statement about the reputation of care homes, about
the reputation of carers. I ask her if she feels alone.

'Yes sometimes you do, do feel very vulnerable.'

A senior walks in and it all becomes too noisy – we have to stop.

(Winston Grove)

Although Diane reported that the work is enjoyable, her enjoyment is
marred by the perceived deprivation of time and concern. Diane's picture
of daily care work is bleak. She talks about being called a black bastard,
remembering excluding notices on shop doors in the sixties, seventies.
She associates the racism she endures at work, and as a younger woman,
with the anti-semitism of the Second World War, of concentration camps.
Diane appears to be conjuring up an unremittingly brutal world, in which
humanity is absent and people are treated as part-objects (Klein, 1952),
receptacles for raging aggression and hatred.

If we track Diane's argument, she begins by talking about being
chastised by the management. Sometimes a resident is very agitated,
and Diane finds herself subjected to racist abuse. She is nonetheless
able to recognise in the residents', and in her own, experience a pain
that is individual and also shared. In doing this, Diane expresses a deep
empathy with a resident's distress, imagining where this might come
from in the past. She says something about the gruelling reality of
day-to-day exposure to racism and how she finds ways to respond. She
goes on to describe an organisational culture that has little response
to these daily encounters with racism other than through formalities
and procedures drained of both practical effect and of the awareness of
human suffering. Organisationally race was ignored as a factor affecting
the caring experience at Winston Grove. This is a powerful example
of someone struggling to make space to think about her work in a

context where the capacity to do so is, at the very least, under increased pressure.

Diane is simultaneously speaking about something else, below the surface, even harder to articulate at an organisational level. Diane talks about a set of experiences that seem to be characterised by systematic and extreme persecution (concentration camps, overt racism, exclusion), by the indifference of those in authority who ought to do something about it (but deal in formalities), and individual isolation and vulnerability in the face of this. This is not to say that the home itself was characterised by systematic persecution. Despite occasional glimpses of something sadistic, it was not a brutal place. However, the content and emotional tone of Diane's comments were shocking and raw, alerting us to the more aggressive unprocessed feelings which were part of life and work at Winston Grove. Speculating, this might have been about the intense anxiety felt in the face of human decay and death, and relatedly the aggressive feelings that such anxiety evokes.

Beyond this, Diane was making an indirect case for locating human pain in a wider socio-historical context. Her pain is current – she feels abused within the home – yet it builds upon past pain, which evokes the history of racism in the UK. Diane flags up one strand of the experience there: that human suffering, and the consequences of history and social circumstance on human suffering, could barely be acknowledged.

Indeed, care home life is often disconnected from the outside, from the current and past historical context. People with dementia rarely know which year they are living in. In that sense, perhaps Diane's narrative says something about human pain, and also about the cut-off experience of living in a care home, where one's identity might be viewed at times one-dimensionally as a subject of daily routinised organisational life. In such a context, people are never fully seen.

For Diane, Winston Grove could be relentless and inhuman. Working there makes her angry, delinquent and vulnerable. Diane's organisation-in-the-mind is characterised by a complex web of persecution and revolt. Even the dog is attempting to uncage himself during her interview.

Work stirs up anxieties, reminding her of 'things that frighten us in cupboards', of unprocessed memories. It is not a homely, safe place. Here time is taken away, through psychic and/or physical death. We are reminded by Diane that in its wake death leaves us with hauntings and haunted people. Unlike Gemma, who represents the aliveness at Winston

Grove – the sometimes manic, triumphant, fight against dying – Diane seems to capture not just death but the cruelty of ending here.

The lack of safety Diane depicts is associated with the mean distribution of time. Where time could support greater humanity for those who are dying, it is instead fought over, a site of one-upmanship. Diane bemoans the fact that her explanations, which take time, are not thought about organisationally. The leadership, in her mind, does not care about her or the people she looks after. Time, or its absence, silences feeling.

Speed and efficiency, concepts often found in new managerialism, and often used as measures against which carers can be assessed, are linked for Diane with bullying, ill-treatment. Her story relates to how she feels those above her do not take the time to listen to her difficulties. Her protestations are not heard, in the same way that the residents who are speeded up are not heard. From her perspective, the care field is riddled with layers and layers of top-down objectifying practice that filters all the way down to the residents. Given the general thread of Diane's argument, it is symptomatic perhaps that a senior carer interrupts her, stopping speech, marking the end of Diane's attempt to be heard. What also became clear, though, as Diane's powerful thoughts and feelings were disrupted, is how easily thinking about race and its effects on the experience of working in the care home was dismissed. Arguably Diane provided evidence for the need of staff teams to be given access to a third, reflective space (Britton, 1989) to process their experiences of the work.

In contrast to Diane, Celia, Bridget, and Gemma's interviews, the organisation-in-the-mind which Ursula depicted provided a modified, less impassioned account, less split in its representation.

URSULA

Ursula works part-time. She seemed neither keen to speak, nor resistant to it. Her physicality and speech seemed to communicate something measured about her. She was statuesque, articulating her words in a considered, unhurried way.

Time was present in what she said in a different way from others. Perhaps the ending of her shift (as well as her part-time role) acted as a boundary for the time she spent talking and for the content.

'I only work here part-time... so the reason I chose actually to be here part-time is to enjoy it... I have noticed that I can actually be a lot more patient than I thought I would be... which has surprised me I have to

say because I didn't think I would be able to be that patient… You get to know a person and you know roughly how they are, what they like, what they don't like. But then again it's all a process. They are going through a process in their mind and it's not always the same, but that's the same with us: we are not always the same. But with someone with dementia it is probably more so.'

Ursula reflects on the many dimensions involved in being human; she has found new dimensions to herself. The care work has led to an experience of expansiveness for her. She is not hemmed in.

'… just take it as it comes really and try and not get set into my own ideas. So yeah, if I'm flexible enough that helps. If I think it has to be done there and then because it's half eleven it might not work. Time is important in a way because it is important in the setting of a care home to a certain extent, but then again it shouldn't be that important to let everything else revolve around a certain set pattern. That is sometimes difficult but there are ways around it.'

Ursula is not denying the very real time constraints, but she herself will not be imprisoned by them. 'Yes, it's the polarity between getting satisfaction of working with people and it being a big challenge at the same time. That's there every day; it's a challenge and also really getting a lot out of what you are doing. If it all goes well and you have a feeling that you have done your best and you have tried to make their experience as positive as you can then the positive side outweighs definitely everything else. But that's not always possible. That's just reality. On a day-to-day basis that's not what you'll experience every day. When there is a shortage of staff and you can't do as much as you would like to and you go home with a feeling that it's not quite that satisfying. But, uh, that's reality.'

(Winston Grove)

Ursula recognises the frustration that timetabling and rigid institutionalised routine bring, but there is some freedom to bend time. Ursula derives pleasure from her job, partially because she works part-time. Perhaps this protects her from the relentlessness of the care work: she implies that she gets time to recuperate from the emotional labour of the work. It seems that this might enable Ursula to manage the uncertainty of working with people with dementia.

Ursula reflects a little on how the work has changed her, and what she has learned from being a carer. Overstretched, as many are, there is undoubtedly less time to be able to reflect like this for full-time workers. This is an interesting formulation because it demonstrates that, with experience and time, she has become more patient and understanding of those in her care. So 'time-in' work is experience for Ursula. Simultaneously, 'time-off' work, through part-time hours, makes it possible for her to consider the care work. Time here relates to space for reflection. Time is about movement and change: she sees the minute-by-minute changes of people with dementia. Ursula does not feel persecuted by the institutional time frame as Diane and Celia do. She seems to tolerate the routines as a marker of contextual reality, while feeling she has enough agency to manipulate time when necessary.

Being pushed for time was not a theme that emerged in talks with staff at Whittinghall. The ratios between care workers and residents were better. The staff team did not seem to challenge the way the home was organised as they did at Winston Grove. There was a greater idealisation of the home, as a family place, seemingly in disconnect with Dorothy's experience there.

The team at Whittinghall was more guarded, as if the organisation itself shied away from in-depth relating and intimacy. Beyond this, Nancy was the only staff member at Whittinghall who explicitly made reference to the notion of time. Time was present, however, in the conversations with the staff team in the sense that meetings were generally cut short. However, although the residents, too, did not point to time as an explicit feature of their experience, the residents at Whittinghall did speak at length, which possibly demonstrated their need for companionship. Let us meet Nancy, Dorothy's keyworker and senior carer.

NANCY AT WHITTINGHALL

Nancy, we know, as Dorothy's keyworker, a senior carer in Huntside unit. She is no more than twenty-five. She has been in the home for up to five years, part of a long-standing team. She worked in another care home before this one, but didn't feel as comfortable there because she felt the team didn't care as much.

No private room is available for interview. Nancy suggests we speak in the lounge. No one is there apart from the stuffed tiger on top of an imposing keyboard. The doors are shut and there are no interruptions. Nancy seems proud of the routines she describes.

'... and then like there is a set routine but if the routine changes, the staff, we are happy to do whatever here... We all like have our own little jobs so we don't need to say, "Oh you go in and do that resident, stay with that resident or this resident on that day." We all know who to help and who to go to at that certain time.'

The routine makes things neat and tidy, like the uniforms the staff wear. There is a logic to this.

'... if we're confused they'll get even more confused... So they'll all be running round not knowing what's going on so we all know what's going on... There are four of us that are always here.' Nancy lists the names of the staff and the days of the week they each work, almost going through the rota; there is always a permanent person on shift. 'Four of us are permanently here and the nurse all the time.'

'We, like, control the unit.' Nancy lets out a laugh and yet this doesn't seem to be a joke. 'We know limits, when to have fun and when not to like be serious and things like that. And we have fun with the residents and they join in... Like when... It's Christmas Day and we all sit down with them and get the Christmas tree out and we open presents together. At least then they know what they are doing. What's going on.'

(Whittinghall)

Nancy and the senior team are in 'control' of the unit, and the way time is ordered. Nancy is not at the mercy of time; she is a time-manager. This bore out in the way that the care staff ensured they took breaks. Nancy and the others always made sure that they were refuelled, leaving the unit during the morning shift.

Time was about order and structure at Whittinghall, something that helped staff keep a distance from the confused temporal spaces of the residents. It is resonant of mothers who find it comforting to create rigid routines for newborns, possibly fearing the pull to slip into baby time.

Nancy had talked about Christmas, symbolising the compartmentalised nature of Whittinghall. Fun is reserved for specific events. The organisation for Nancy is rational, unconfused, neat but lacking in spontaneity. It is as if the uncertainty that dementia arouses doesn't have a place there.

This mirrored the staff's response to Dorothy, who had a clear physical space in the organisation between two red velvet chairs in the corridor, but whose complex, muddled needs were sometimes painfully overlooked. Although the home had won accolades for its dementia care, the staff team was young and, in a manner that was perhaps developmentally appropriate, took more time to relate to one another. Sadly this often meant avoiding the residents.

Residents' relation to time

The residents at Winston Grove considered time from the point of view of past lives. Attempts were made to integrate former senses of selves, with whom they were now in the present moment. There was a real need to spend time bearing witness to their stories, often evoked with a real emotional eloquence.

Maude, who we will meet shortly, used the time to play; and Sue used time to mourn.

Maude is a woman in her eighties, who had enjoyed music all her life. We are in her bedroom. Maude surrounds herself with all manner of cuddly toys – large teddies, small bees, and tiny ducks, and her favourite, Winnie the Pooh. Maude introduces every toy, and theoretically thoughts of transitional objects came to the fore (Winnicott, 1971; Stephens et al, 2012). At the end of our conversation, she says, 'Oh I'm delighted that you have taken an interest in the little things, you know.'

'Everyone that comes in, you know, they're all young children and I let them just say hello… and all the rest of it to enjoy the short time they are here with you.' It's clear Maude feels at home here, at least in her bedroom. 'I don't pine for, you know, or wish I was where I had been so… what was this one? They all have a bit of character. It's so silly but I can't think. I know that's Winnie. There is a story about Winnie, a book, so that could be of some interest.' She laughs, then notes her confusion. 'Now I don't know what I'm doing actually… He seems very familiar to me… Oh excuse me.' I pick up Winnie. 'Oh you clever girl, you. I want it to go all the way down here. That's my photograph. These are all my little precious things. They're nice for… if children come in I let them play with them for a little while.' Maude continues, each personality in her room noted. It's a lively place. 'Individually they are quite interesting. That's Scotty. This is

Quack Quack.' She repositions Scotty and Quack Quack so that they look like they are talking. 'There they are having a chat.' As she and I are. 'I feel that they all belong... I don't know if you want a chair or something. I've been collecting those little things that are on the windowsill there... they... they open and you can put something in. It's interesting. I'm free to come and go which is very nice. That's Winnie there. I'm dedicated to them... it's lovely going around saying, "oh you know, the time I looked after you and you were almost talking to me".

(Winston Grove)

Talking with Maude was baffling because we didn't follow an unfolding linear narrative. She flitted, or free associated, from one significant object in her room to another. But the emotional content told a tale about what it was like to be at Winston Grove for Maude in that present moment.

She had a warm, welcoming room, filled to the brim with friendly faces on photographs and on soft toys. It was as if this environment fed into a secure internal structure, or bolstered one, already at home where Maude could be Maude, where she was reminded of music, play, and inviting encounters with parents, partner, and children. It was not that Maude dwelled on time, or felt she was missing out on time, but rather that she appreciated time to be and to play with her figures and trinkets. Time allowed her to breathe further life into this mingling of past and present from which she could draw strength. Time was generous, opening up the space for sharing and the possibility of constructing a joint experience; a bit like her little boxes, treasures could be found there.

At the end of one of the bingo games with Gemma, Maude had been singing 'Amazing Grace'. It had been a very evocative moment where spontaneous self-expression had been tolerated. At Winston Grove, she felt able to be herself. She had not been bothered about the lack of prizes for bingo; the prize for Maude was being given time to sing a song that brought her back to herself.

An oscillation between past and present selves seems to be a feature of dementia, very much related to temporality. As we will see from Sue's account, a new resident at Winston Grove, there was a powerful need for her to make connections with the past, as if this would provide her with some safety as she faced the uncertainty, unfamiliarity, of a new life at Winston Grove. Here Sue was in new surroundings, following a lengthy hospital admission. We see her grappling with the anxiety of where she is and how she has come to be so far from home (her childhood home).

Sue, a woman in her seventies, originally from Wales, had only been living in the home for a fortnight. She has long loose hair and glasses. Her face is gentle and she speaks so very softly. She has no relatives close by, and has been discharged from hospital following a fall. Her room is sparse, no identifying features, no pictures or photos or signs of a life before.

Sue is happy to talk. She had been sitting in a lounge, quietly with other residents, silent. She spends much time looking out of the window. She has just been saying that she needs to get back to the small village in Wales where she grew up. She has talked about her school and church, about returning to Mum on the bus.

'It's very interesting… I've never had such a type of a reception from anyone. What do you think we could do? Oh cariad ('love' in Welsh).' She is looking out of the window. 'This uh got a ball. Old. By the beach.' She is someplace else. 'We would go for walks. With the dog. Then we get there. I wouldn't know how to get there, no. Very sad [Sue is crying] when people disappear.' She takes deep breaths. She clasps her hands tightly together and starts to look out of the window again. 'That's where the university… The time that used to go.'

(Winston Grove)

Sue was in contact with her emotional world and the profound experience of loss she was undergoing. She had travelled back to a period in her life when she needed school, chapel and Mum. It became clear how unfamiliar the residential home was, as she yearned to get back to a place among people to whom she belonged. She spoke for a long time, tearful and in mourning.

Sue's relationship to time held within it a paradox: she knew that school and friends from Wales were a 'long time ago', yet she felt driven to find a real bus outside that would bridge a gap between her memories and her current position. We discussed bus routes and what she would say to people she missed. This allowed her to return to a past-time and act it out in the present. Though it was painful for Sue to summon up figures from her past, especially her mother, she needed someone to be present to the changes she was facing internally and in her immediate environment. Sue was able to express gratitude for my being with her, and this in turn made me want to spend time with her. This kind of co-affecting seemed to take place among residents and care staff throughout the home, and yet this kind of intimacy is barely recognised in the work.

And yet being with someone as they attempt to understand that times and people past are 'disappearing' is both a privilege and a hardship for staff.

At Whittinghall, time and the impact of loss were more pronounced. This seemed to fit with my view of Whittinghall as a place where residents often withdrew into themselves towards death.

Time was so heavy in Whittinghall, partially because Dorothy was always positioned in the corridor opposite a large clock, as if time had been suspended and nothing seemed to change. She frequently cried out 'Tuesday, Tuesday, Tuesday', or 'Thursday, Thursday, Thursday', reading out the sign on the wall that told her what day it was. It was as if she was holding on tightly to some kind of temporal reality, yet it seemed simultaneously to be a cause of anxiety rather than comfort, as if nothing felt real. Similarly, when Dorothy read the clock, this made her feel alone and confused, perhaps a sense that time was moving on as she stayed still, all by herself. The following two vignettes evoke the sense of the panic that time seemed to generate in Dorothy:

Dorothy starts to close her eyes and bends her head down into her chest. Nancy says that Dorothy won't take her medication at 7am and is taking it later now. Dorothy is presenting the team with challenges. This is making her more tired. Yesterday she put Dorothy to bed at 4pm and only woke her up for her tea at night, then she went back to sleep. She said she thought that if she put her to bed now she would just keep sleeping. Dorothy's eyes open up again, a contradiction. It wasn't clear whether Dorothy's medication related to some of her more 'disruptive' behaviours, her agitation, demanding calls. Whatever it was Nancy seemed to think that it was knocking Dorothy out at times.

From the lounge a man emerges. Nancy jumps up and asks the man where his frame is, protectively. She asks him to stand still for a moment and she runs into the lounge, retrieving his frame. Dorothy watches this with wide open eyes, then turns her head back to the nurses' station. 'That time,' she says looking at the clock.

Being seated each week opposite the clock on the wall above the nurses' station meant that time was ever present here. It seemed to slow down.

The longer hand on the clock would tick on, moments ebbing away, time stretching out in the corridor. This made it seem as though Dorothy was always waiting for the clock to stop, for something to happen, for night-time to come and take her. The clock, coupled with Dorothy's rare movement, stirred up thoughts of Godot, of the relentless futility of existence. This was hard to sit with.

(Whittinghall)

Dorothy wants to cut off. She herself is sleeping more, which the staff understand to be an effect of the medication. It is as if the sheer boredom of being in the same place every day, with minimal human contact, is forcing her into retreat. Sometimes it is as if Dorothy is in solitary confinement. Here she is again, now left with just echoes of her own sound:

Dorothy is sitting in her usual position opposite the nurses' station, between two red velvet armchairs. She is wearing a beige gilet and a brown polo neck jumper, with brown trousers. She looks smart, very smart. There are no members of staff around. She raises up her right hand as if to wave, but instead makes her hand into the bird's head, moving it up and down. A fledgling in need of feeding, a silhouette, shadowy figure, in a puppet show, outlines to be filled in. How do we get to know Dorothy?

'Hello, hello, hello,' she says.

Another resident with very big glasses is moving in front of Dorothy, on her zimmer frame.

It is noisy in the corridor, as one of the care assistants is hoovering. 'What's he doing, he doing, he doing?' says Dorothy. 'Noisy, very noisy, noisy,' says Dorothy. She looks at the table to the left of her. There is a beaker and a glass of orange juice there. She looks away, moving her feet a little on the wheelchair footrests. 'Tuesday, Tuesday, Tuesday,' she says repeatedly, as if this one thing that at least feels concrete. We have been here before and we wonder if this is one way that helps Dorothy to feel less at sea. There is something Sisyphean in this existence, and the rock... it feels as though it is getting heavier as time passes on.

She notices a clock and tries to tell the time. 'I have no idea, no idea, no idea.' Perhaps time is standing still.

'Wendy, Wendy, Wendy,' she shouts louder, raising up her hand in the bird-like shape to be noticed. A nurse and the care assistant have a

conversation in the corridor about slings and hoists; Dorothy gives up, shaking her head and then placing it in her hands. The nurse disappears. The care assistant puts the hoover back on. 'I can't hear a thing,' says Dorothy.

(Whittinghall)

An experience of lost objects was palpable in observations with Dorothy. This was also true of Evie, who was sometimes seated next to her in the corridor:

Dorothy starts to try to pull her purple jumper further down over her trousers, as if she is rearranging herself, then stops. She looks into the distance, then turns, 'Where are the others?' She cuts a lone figure out here in the corridor. 'I'm not sure where the others are.' Someone is lost; Nancy has just gone. Dorothy bends her head slightly and then puts her head in her hands, staying there some time.

'Wendy,' she calls out, hauntingly.

'Wendy won't be long,' says the nurse behind the station, popping her head around to try to make contact with Dorothy. Dorothy nods.

'Where are the others?' she asks into the distance, seeming to have heard the nurse.

'They'll all be back for lunchtime.'

'Wendy,' says Dorothy. The nurse's response hasn't quelled the panic.

'She won't be long,' says the nurse, this time a disembodied voice.

Dorothy swallows; tears form a little in her eyes.

The manager, Amy, is in the distance, showing someone around the rooms in the home. 'Hello,' she says to me. 'Hope it's okay that I have left you with Nancy.' And now I have been left with Dorothy. A handing over here and there.

(Whittinghall)

The experience of lost objects and of being left alone to work things out also emerged in discussions with a male resident, Dr Jesmond. In his conversation with me, he also suggests, albeit implicitly, that he expects a more timely response from the staff team. Other issues were flagged up in this conversation, around choice and control, for example, but for now we will concentrate on Dr Jesmond's sense that the staff team is wasting time and that he has a perpetual experience of waiting, of time passing by.

Dr Jesmond spoke for twenty minutes. He explained that his stay in the home was a temporary one, although in actuality it was permanent. He said that his wife visited daily to have lunch with him, although this was questionable. He looked physically very fit and had only one or two grey hairs. He was a domineering presence, a bit of an anomaly in the home. He was very keen to make sure wine was available for lunch, even though alcohol only appeared on special occasions.

The presence of the care marketplace found its way into the interview with Dr Jesmond, the only resident with whom I spoke who had a sense of himself as a consumer.

'... a good day, everything goes smoothly... the food's all right; the wine's all right; the service is all right [he has a little chuckle]. You know it's... that's all it is. Do things go well or not? I suppose it's just the same as anywhere else in the country. Yeah, you know, um, I think on the whole the service is very good...

But at the moment I don't know where my wife is... she's somewhere around and, uh, I quite like, I like getting in touch with her for the, the meal, or I'm not quite sure, the supper.

Well, yes, unless there's a special arrangement been made for her by somebody else in the building, saying well we've made an arrangement for you to go to such and such... and on those occasions she quite likes it if they sort of say we've got your husband to come along too... so they tell me [he breaks out into laughter]. It's just that if I'm out all of the time I don't see her [there is a strange noise in the background, like building works]... we'll just have to wait and see. But um I think on the whole it all goes reasonably well but speak to somebody who's not very pleased and see what they say.

That's all I was doing in actual fact. My main objective because um I knew that the food... They have a kitchen for that...

So I think that, touch wood, it's probably going to go all right today. But you're never 100 per cent sure until the time comes and I think well, "Why aren't we having this or that or the other...?" and then trying to find somebody who I think should be responsible for that particular element of the meal, the drinks or whatever, and then I try to tap away and say "What's happening?" and if I'm lucky they'll say "It's all going ahead as planned" [he laughs] and if it's not they look at you blankly and say, "What are you talking about?" [He laughs.]

That is very frustrating because I think to myself... I am talking to them about their job and they should come back immediately and say,

"This is what we are doing and this is how it's going" and as far as I'm concerned it's all going well. But you know life is like that… it's like that… and in the big outside world too. I find it very difficult, you see, I can't predict some of the problems. You conclude usually that some idiot in the team has done something very silly… [sighs] and you wish they hadn't… Okay well… little time to waste. So I'm just sort of hanging around, waiting for the next hopeful stage in the procedure… Which I thought ought to be… a little wine… not necessarily handed to people but at least a little bit of wine in the area… so when we need it we know where it is… accessible.'

(Whittinghall)

Dr J is holding on to the idea of the availability wine. Getting it would be a victory in this comfortable place which nonetheless confuses him. Having lost his wife, he needs to try to take control of something, something that reminds him of the person he once was, a man who talked about memberships to some of the elite local clubs and often had wine at his lunchtime meals.

As time moves on, into older age, it brings with it losses. In some cases, like Dorothy's, there was little or no opportunity to think about them, and what they meant to her. Evie, also resident in Huntside unit, was also left with the gap that 'Johnny' had left. It felt unbearable to witness these two women cry out for the disappeared, as if they were forced into re-experiencing an absence over and over again.

Dorothy is sitting in her usual position beside the coffee table to her left and a red velvet armchair to her right. Another woman, small, thin and frail-looking, is in the chair to the left of her. She is slouched down in the armchair to Dorothy's right. One of the male carers is sitting next to her, drinking from his bottle of juice. 'I can see you, I can see you,' smiles Dorothy.

The woman next to her has her eyes closed and starts to call out, 'Johnny, Johnny, Johnny.'

The male carer starts to push himself up out of the chair. A call for me to take up his place? He walks away into the lounge area.

Dorothy is watching the nurses' station. A male nurse in navy blue is filling out files. 'They're not doing anything, nothing at all,' Dorothy says critically.

(Whittinghall)

This was one of many times where Evie was observed calling out for someone from a time gone by, and no answer came. It was common for several members of staff to be present and to have time available to respond. Nonetheless Evie and Dorothy were denied their time, minutes which could have been used to more adequately reassure them or to find something out about these lost figures that haunted their everyday lives.

At Winston Grove the way that time was treated was contradictory and multi-layered. Time was hankered after by many carers, as if it might be a magic wand, a way into better care and relating. For the staff at Winston Grove, greater access to time signified the possibility of making contact with the residents, and was also related to carving out a position of greater authority (though not formally in terms of role) within the organisation. The time pre- and post-austerity was also thought about. Carers like Celia and Diane presented a real split between care practices now and then, so much so that the level of reward in the care work felt increasingly out of reach to them. Arguably this felt like an occupational death.

In Whittinghall there was a quiet closing down among the staff team, possibly a defence against being infected by dementia. Perhaps this represented a split between the time of youth and the time of old age. Time at Whittinghall belonged to the workers, as they ordered it into easy-to-manage routines. There was little place in this orderliness to recognise the confused temporal spaces of the residents with dementia, which was very real.

Although Nancy made a lot of effort with Dorothy and showed signs of real fondness for her, she was able to break off quite cruelly, as other members of the team did. Time seemed to belong to the staff, who found ways to keep living by being together and retreating to spaces, psychic and physical, unavailable to the residents, like the nurses' station.

Among the residents the sense of loss (lost objects, lost sense of self, the need to mourn) was palpable in both homes, though Daphne and Maude seemed to represent the possibility of sharing time with others that facilitated an integration of past and present times, and of inner and outer realities. No doubt the older people also enjoyed time with carers, and others, to share experience. This replicated my experience in both homes where encounters were often slow-moving and involved real tenderness.

The dyadic relationship between mother and infant springs to mind here: the desire to feel contained and held is vital in dementia care. Considering, too, that many people with dementia return to earlier periods in their lives, yet unconsciously might be in touch with the fact that they are faced with greater losses, or un-developments, rather than gains, the need for carers who have time, or who feel able to share their time, seems to be a pressing issue.

Understanding time

As I have already described, one particular feature of the thinking around time at Winston Grove was a pervasive splitting. Bridget, the housekeeper, Celia, the longest-serving carer, Diane, the carer, and Gemma, the activities co-ordinator, differentiated good caregivers from bad according to the way that they treated time. Among all of them there was a sense that those carers who stretched, slowed down time, were doing care 'right' by the residents. These four members of staff claimed that they adapted their pace to the residents'. Bridget and Gemma saw this as a privilege of their roles, while Celia and Diane felt they were making a conscious protest against organisational time pressures in order to offer the best care they could give. All distinguished themselves from 'bad' carers on the grounds that they 'made time' for residents as human beings. In Armstrong's (2005) terms, they resisted the punctuation of interpersonal space that time-as-task-management represented.

For Bridget, carers were at a disadvantage because of the routinised task-focused structure of the home. This meant that the speed at which carers worked precluded them from getting to know the residents. Gemma spoke of the carers with a mix of frustration and empathy. Gemma understood that carers hurried time along so that physical jobs could be done. However she was also critical that they were, as she saw it, both unable and unwilling to slow down to enjoy and benefit from the social, emotional, component of the work, which she felt she represented for the organisation as the activities co-ordinator. Gemma's ambivalent account demonstrated that there was some capacity organisationally to hold in place contradictory understandings and feelings, that the defence employed was not always an obvious splitting.

Celia and Diane, both carers, did not feel at a loss in the way Gemma described. They railed against perceived time constraints and avoided succumbing to a 'hotel model', 'conveyor belt' style of relating. Their protests meant that they understood the complexities and needs of the residents, allowing them to do a better job. The divide was not between overly busy, hands-on care staff and those with time to relate to residents, but between those staff holding fast to 'person-centred' approaches to care and, as they saw it, those assimilated to the new 'hotel' model promoted by a management needing to do more with less. As a denigrated mode of caring, the 'hotel model' practices were located in other members of the team. For Celia, temporary workers offered care in this way and, for Diane, these practices belonged to those who considered themselves efficient workers (the 'super, super' people).

For both women, the treatment of time seemed to be a vehicle through which certain organisational power dynamics played out, of the type that Benjamin (2006) describes as doer-done-to relating. With Diane and Celia, an unspoken power dynamic during the course of our conversations was palpable. In my counter-transference with Celia, I felt small, inexperienced, unknowing about frontline care. I sat on the edge of a bed listening to her intently, as if she knew things that I knew nothing about. I felt strangely infantile in relation to her dominant voice. With Diane, the power dynamic may have played out around which one of us understood what was really happening in the care context. You may remember Diane pointing out that she might not be the right person with whom to speak. There was also a power dynamic, I thought, around our racial differences, which I will discuss at the end of this chapter (and which I barely addressed during the course of the interview in the same way that the home avoided thinking about people's experiences of race and racism). I wondered how much a sense of guilt about my own privileged, white, educated researcher status had fed into me, unconsciously inverting the power dynamics that are often present in society at large.

With both Celia and Diane, and to a certain extent Bridget, I had a sense of being inadequate as a researcher, and I wondered whether this was how they felt in relation to the way that care work[13] is generally undervalued. Relatedly, in the counter-transference with all three, I had a strong sense that I needed to give them time to express their thoughts and experience, affording them an authority and agency that perhaps felt

13 Considered low-skilled, often carried out by women considered working class (Gallagher, *Guardian 2017*, n.p.)

out of reach societally and within the organisation. In Gemma, too, the question of knowing and authority materialised, when she asked me if she was on the right track. Returning to the organisation-in-the-mind, it is quite possible that these interviews provided me with varying pieces of intelligence about the emotional reality of Winston Grove, particularly around a sense of helplessness associated with not being heard, an experience that may also have resonated with the residents.

My feelings of not-knowing vis-à-vis Celia, Diane, and Bridget, and a feeling of knowing in relation to Gemma suggested that there was something known in the emotional and imaginal life of the organisation, but which had eluded formulation (Armstrong, 2005, p. 51). In relation to all four participants, this thing which was known yet couldn't be thought about was the precariousness of occupational authority in times of austerity, also perhaps the divisions of power associated with class and race. It was telling that with all four women I felt that I really needed to give them time, listen to their stories. Although the domineering voices of Bridget and Celia were possible reactions to my presence as a bearer of academic privilege and knowledge, I suspect they were also striking back at the loss of being valued in their role/s.

This all begged a further question, which was not necessarily just bound up with the insecurities brought about by austerity. I wondered to myself 'Why was it important for workers to feel a degree of precariousness in their roles?', and, through a sort of institutional projective identification, 'Why should I feel so unknowing as a researcher?' It seemed to me that it was highly likely that these vulnerable experiences mirrored the experience of increasingly dependent people with dementia, reliant as they were on a system that was, despite the optimism of the National Dementia Strategy (2009), itself more unstable and uncertain than before.

Diane and Celia had framed their interview around the wider care crisis, brought about by austerity politics. Bridget also feared an occupational death, a real sense of being undervalued in the work she did. It seemed, then, that the splitting that all women engendered was brought about by a harsh, austere reality that fostered this kind of psychic response among members of society, particularly among those most likely to be penalised in relation to class, gender, and race. By undermining certain segments of the population (the elderly population and those who care for them being one branch), a need to reassert, to find power and voice seemed to be imperative – in the face of possible social and occupational annihilation.

SPLITTING: A TIME TO CARE

It is worth reiterating that, in the minds of staff at Winston Grove, speed was equated to routinisation, inhumanity. A slower pace was seen as supporting human agency. Despite the fact that there was some evidence of an unrealistically demanding organisation-at-work at Winston Grove, there was room for carer discernment in the use of time. Even though there was not a rigidly strict protocol around time, time was at a premium. Indeed, stretching time for residents even came at a personal cost to staff members (leaving later, a build-up of care planning work, and so forth).

In terms of the organisational culture of Winston Grove, the neat black-and-white split of good and bad care could be understood from a Kleinian perspective. Diane and Celia used 'making time' to communicate a psychic split related to a resistance to organisational change; Bridget's splitting seemed to be around the care home hierarchies, which distinguished between roles, and may have related both to class and race; and finally Gemma's was seen in terms of status distinctions between peers. Kleinian (1946) explanations on the psychic mechanisms involved in split states of mind is helpful here. It is possible to recognise patterns of relating, and thinking, between individuals which create organisational cultures where a paranoid-schizoid functioning exists.

The splitting among the staff team was a response to the wider austerity agenda, and to the position one found oneself in within the organisation. It is also possible that the staff were reacting to, and were receptacles for, the splitting pervasive in the client group in a care home. Klein recognised that there is an ongoing potential across the life course for the emergence of destructive states of mind in the face of persecutory anxiety. Indeed, people with dementia often feel persecuted by the condition itself.

As Froggett (2002) notes, in a human care context, 'welfare agencies, hospitals and schools are very familiar with splitting in clients who rage against a particular worker while idealising another' (p. 37). As I have said, this kind of splitting was noticed in both homes.

TIME TO INTEGRATE LIFE AND DEATH

Chaya, Gemma and Bridget, at Winston Grove, were often idealised by residents. Similarly, Nancy was by Dorothy, at Whittinghall. Other carers, such as Diane, were denigrated and disliked. This allowed residents to protect certain carers from their more destructive feelings, seeing in the good objects of care (Gemma, Chaya, Nancy) the possibility for rescue. Some members of staff arguably became the receptacles of aggressive projections and others housed all the good feeling. This made the organisation appear to be a split unintegrated place. Often those staff who were idealised were those able to push aside the task and give their time over to the residents. Diane, who claimed she valued residents' time over her own, was sometimes painfully slow to serve up lunch. This enforced sense of waiting may have made her a target for bad-object attacks. We may remember how attached Dorothy was to Nancy until Nancy began to take an increasing number of breaks, then a holiday. It was after this point, when Nancy had less time, that she was no longer such a good object. A weaning of sorts, in dementia care, is unlikely to generate the kind of recognition Benjamin (2009) might describe.

The same was true of the way staff members appreciated some residents over others. At times, it was as if a sort of love-hate feedback loop was in play. However, there were also movements out of paranoid-schizoid states into states of a more ambivalent depressive nature (Klein, 1937). The latter was particularly evident when carers reflected on the fear of damaging those they looked after – for instance, Nancy's moving reflections on Dorothy's potential death, explaining that she would have to leave Huntside, the unit for elderly frail residents, once Dorothy died. Bridget also talked about losing her patience with a resident, and feeling guilty for months after. In both homes, though, there was a sense that time for this kind of reflection was inadequate, that more was needed.

Influenced by Freud, Klein's (1946) ideas give us an understanding of the experience of dementia which is rooted partially in the instinctual. For someone post-verbal, there is arguably a movement back towards more unfiltered experience, where the drives – particularly the death drive, we may surmise – regain power and hold over individuals. In a care context, anxieties about existence easily leak into psychic and organisational space. The death drive is a hugely powerful internal primitive tendency, arguably on the borderline with the psyche and the soma, always in conflict with life drives and the need for connection, love. The split between notions of good and bad care are quite possibly responses to the anxieties aroused by such conflicts, likely to be heightened in an end-of-life context. There might have been a fantasy at Winston Grove about which members of staff were able to keep people psychically, socially, physically, alive. The way that stretched time was valued over momentary encounters may have been viewed symbolically as a way to stave off death, although it was clear that joining residents at their own pace was vital for connection.

The idea of death/life drives can be linked to the very real need for time to care. When staff take time to care, the effect for the residents might amount to a certain re-fusing of the death and life drives, enabling them to *be*. For the staff there may also be a kind of re-fusing of the drives in the face of the time-driven pressures of the organisation, under austerity conditions, which generate feelings of 'dying' occupationally. Unrealistic time pressures on the staff disrupt the capacity to care, one consequence of which is that the drives for both residents and staff become prone to diffusion and the subsequent organisational splitting that follows.

At large, the organisational splitting at Winston Grove was undoubtedly in the service of a paranoid-schizoid organisational functioning – the desire to retreat into bad and good part-objects (Klein, 1946; 1952), creating entrenched positions to avoid thinking about the pain of being personally close to the dementing and the dying. Thinking about the residents' precariousness and fragility proved to be intensely difficult because a sense of occupational precariousness was also around. It had been reported that in former times the training budget allowed for Alzheimer's Society training and dementia care diplomas. There had also once been a visiting psychologist who discussed residents on a case-by-case basis with members of staff. None of this was currently available.

The split between notions of good and bad care was a multi-layered response to neoliberalism, to austerity agendas and also towards the hierarchies within the organisation. This split also related to an existential fear aroused by working around death and dying. Certainly for Gemma, less inclined to protest against austerity (although she did mention corners being cut), she saw herself as central to maintaining the life of the home. However, in terms of day-to-day care practice her role was peripheral, and perhaps she felt guilty that she could claim time to play. Bridget also carved out an important position, which related to her taking time to get to know people, all in contrast to her lowly position within the hierarchy.

TIME TO MOURN

We might also speculate that the loss of past approaches to care, which Celia talked about at length, and where greater solidarity within the team was remembered, might cause anger that, undigested, could get located in different places and people within the organisation. This is interesting because there was not really space for any form of mourning to be done. Relatedly Froggett (2002) makes the point that,

> The paranoid-schizoid position is essentially a timeless one in which the present is split off from the past and future alike and only the feelings that belong to the here-and-now can be entertained... They deny past experience and rewrite history in terms of the present.

(p. 39)

At Winston Grove, there was a capacity to remember the past, to remember care practice as it had once been, but being able to make the link between the current sadness, anger, and this loss proved difficult. By keeping the two apart – *this is now, that was then* – there was a sense that, organisationally, a limit had been set to further thinking, enquiry. Mourning and reflecting on mourning may well have created a bridge between these two historical points in time that may have provided insights into the experiential reality of workers, and relatedly allowed for greater empathy with the temporal, cognitive, physical, and material losses that the residents were undergoing. It is not to say that the organisation-in-the-mind at Winston Grove was entirely split, but rather that paranoid-schizoid functioning was a large feature of it.

The dementia care field is often in the grip of moment-by-moment affective states. The past is not often thought about, reflectively, but nonetheless it comes to inhabit the present, an unprocessed spectral influence. The dementia care context is in some ways a timeless context, partially because people with dementia live through the immediacy of their emotions, cognitive function often inadequate to the task of thinking about feelings. It is quite possible that, without thinking spaces written into organisational practice, staff members also become drawn into this non-reflective present moment.

The ultimate consequence of the splitting meant that the more enriching, generative possibilities of coming together and re-imagining the primary task of the organisation stayed out of reach. It meant that the primary task was constantly being interpreted, understood, and misunderstood at the level of the individual worker, in part because the leadership was also operating in a split way. This confusion was both personally burdensome and ethically challenging. On many levels, this allowed for the level of anarchy in Winston Grove that made the organisation both exhilarating and muddled. The immediate management, as represented by Elaine, was also anxious about the economic climate, and about having to care for an increasingly dependent client group despite the mounting cuts to resources. Rather than think this through, Elaine subversively joked about sneaking a horse into the garden without the knowledge of her senior management team.

It is possible that, having felt under attack by local and national government, Winston Grove had no inclination to enter discussions with their senior management team (possibly regarded as the mouthpiece for austerity) and to negotiate. Perhaps the organisational splitting was employed in the service of a rebellious protest, seen as necessary. It is possible that the team believed no amount of thinking/talking time would remedy the reality of slashed budgets and more intense time pressures, that only actions that would have an immediate impact on the lives of people at Winston Grove mattered.

Having said that, there was capacity for thinking at Winston Grove, as represented in the part-time care worker, Ursula, who deployed a depressive level of functioning (Klein, 1949). She was able to manage something of the uncertainty of working with people with dementia, neither prone to idealising Winston Grove nor denigrating it. This could be seen in her understanding of both the values of temporal routines and simultaneously the need to bend them. Ursula had not been in the home as long as carers such as Diane and Celia, and possibly this gave her less of an impetus to split between the good past and the bad present. Instead, since she had little to compare it to, she was able to see both the bad and good aspects of the present. Although Ursula's was a reasonably isolated voice, there was some room organisationally to consider the imperfect reality of the contemporary care field. With a structured thinking space, this would have allowed greater engagement with the senior management team, the opportunity to express a range of views.

Whittinghall seemed to have a long way to go in terms of 'making time' to reflect upon the paradoxical aspects of the work, and the sheer volume of feeling associated with those losing their minds. Representative of this difficulty with thinking was the fact that my longest conversation with a care worker was only thirteen minutes. Time to process the worker experience was not valued. Around the theme of time, there did seem to be a process of splitting at work. However, this played out in a very different way at Whittinghall.

My own counter-transference towards staff at Whittinghall was one of irritation. I wondered if this was related to a broader organisational irritation about staff time being interrupted by demands of the residents. I realised I could not express my irritation, and started to imagine that this may have expressed a passive-aggressive stance towards dependent others. Staff were anxious that time for themselves was not interrupted, cut short by the demands of the residents. The organisation-in-the-mind that I registered, through my counter-transference response, was one that cut itself off to the feelings of, and talking with, those facing one final temporal cutting-off. The lack of conversations with staff represented on some levels the reality that there was little time to think.

Nancy's interview demonstrated that time belonged to the workers. It was ordered, controlled by them. As she said, '...there is a set routine but if the routine changes, the staff, we are happy to do whatever... We all know who to help and who to go to at that certain time.' Nancy listed the staff on shift and went through the rota. The clarity of the routine, we might surmise, ensured that the muddle and confusion of dementia would not get into the staff team, protecting them from coming into contact with their messy feelings. There was something deadening about the routinised nature of Whittinghall, which seemed to prevent the freedom of human interaction. By compartmentalising time, there was less chance of an encounter with the frightening experiences of dementia. Generally, at Whittinghall, there was a chasm of a split between the workers and the people with dementia. Time, which belonged to the former group, held more value organisationally than the latter. This possibly communicated something about the developmental position of the young staff team, where time to live took precedence over time to disintegrate and die. We might begin to conceive of a divide where the life and death drives had not been integrated. This reflects a wider societal split, at least in Western cultures, between youth and age, the turning a blind eye to an experience of ageing which is debilitating and difficult.

POTENTIAL SPACE: A TIME TO PLAY

Winnicott emphasises moments where there is a simultaneous inter-subjective creation and discovery of psychic states. This takes place in a space, neither wholly inner nor outer.

Play seemed to offer the possibility of a meeting point between worker and resident experience, of the type that was often absent at

Whittinghall. As Nancy had pointed out, with reference to Christmas Day, pleasure and fun were scheduled there. Arguably a different use of time at Whittinghall, that might have enabled moments of off-rota connection, is worth considering via the Winnnicottian concept of play, a notion through which interesting insights into the organisational cultures of each home emerge.

In Winnicottian terms the capacity to play leads to creative experiences that preserve the sense that 'life is worth living' (Winnicott, 1971, cited in Borden, p. 31). Creative living is about interacting with the world and the environment, with others in and through the fullness of one's paradoxes. This is in counterpoint to engaging with others inauthentically through a false-self carapace. Play is a spontaneous, creative act that allows each of us to make contact with ourselves and with others in an unashamedly truthful way. Playing paves the way for an exploration of experience in which inner psychic reality meets with the realities of others, through a potential space free of judgement. Following play, it is possible that we are able to rediscover a true self, into which we can relax. Winnicott believed (Borden, 1998) that this true self exists before the onset of object relating. Maternal care either hindered or supported its (true self) evolution. Play seems vital in dementia care, since it helps people to return to a place in which they can recreate and rediscover something of their very being. It seems perhaps paradoxical that in a context where people are confused, and where some are dying, play is an important source of expression. However, moments of play in both care homes undoubtedly led to helpful communication and psychological sustenance.

A lack of play involves a relationship with external reality based on compliance. The following quote resonates with the experience of being at Whittinghall, where daily life, as seen through Dorothy's experience, had taken on a Beckettian quality:

> ... the world and its details being recognised but only as something to be fitted in with or demanding adaptation. Compliance carries with it a sense of futility for the individual and is associated with the idea that nothing matters and that life is not worth living.
>
> (Winnicott, 1971, p. 65, cited in Borden, 1998, p. 31)

In his book on Winnicott's life, Adam Phillips (2007) highlights the consequences of a lack of play in an analytic session, suggesting that without time to play a meeting becomes dogmatic and compliant. In terms of Whittinghall, an organisation absent of play may be held to account for the same thing. Indeed, residents were far less likely to become troublesome or to be expressive at Whittinghall: those who were (Dorothy) would be restrained (the brakes on her wheelchair were clamped tight) or medicated (her sleepiness). We might imagine that in an institution anxious to do things correctly, following policy to the letter, there may be less capacity to play. Play involves the sharing of unconscious, disorderly spaces, and this may feel too risky in a procedurally run care home.

Winston Grove, on the other hand, found time to offer moments of spontaneous play as well as the structured play that Gemma represented, which sometimes led to free-flowing play too. It stands to reason that, if we follow Winnicott's line of argument, the residents there were able to move in and out of different versions of themselves, even rebelling against the time demands of the staff team. It is entirely possible that one of the reasons that the staff team were so much more conscious of the value of the residents' time was because, through play, some residents still communicated a joy in living.

For dementia care, Klein's work on the noisier drives and states of mind is invaluable, but we also need Winnicott, particularly his detailed exploration of environmental provisions. A mother making time for play is a mother that supports the development of the capacity to *be* authentically in the world; in dementia care terms, one wonders if an organisation willing to make time to play is able to support older people to be themselves without recourse to feelings of shame, or under pressure to conform to the demands of the organisation.

Winnicott's ideas take us on the developmental trajectory of the child from dependence to relative dependence, through to independence, and the move from unintegrated states to integrated and sometimes disintegrated ones, from which, all being well in early development, we can recover. Dementia takes a person to an increasingly disintegrated state, so part of the work involved in dementia care relates to facilitating moments of reintegration. It is in play, linked to the notion of a transitional space, that people might be able, in relation to others, to experience their authentic selves – even in a state of dementia. In a transitional space, where there is an opportunity to experience connection and separateness with others (often through transitional objects, both *me* and *not-me*), a person with dementia might be embarking on an inverse developmental trajectory to the infant. Soft toys, musical toys, dolls, were used by many residents in Winston Grove, a place where mother was often mentioned. Daphne herself spent one observation moving a doll into a more comfortable sitting position (page 165). As Winnicott notes,

> The [transitional] object represents the infant's transition with being merged with the mother to a state of being in relation to the mother as something outside and separate.
>
> (Winnicott, 2005, p. 19)

Playing, particularly through the use of transitional objects, might at times serve to indicate that a person with dementia is un-forming gradually, making the journey back eventually to a mother (and to the womb). Play provides a space for growth more than knowing; in dementia care, a transitional space is possibly one in which adaptation to, and moments of reintegration on, a precarious journey can take place.

Winston Grove was a place where play opened up a potential space (Winnicott, 1971, p. 72) where staff and residents were able in the moment to be themselves. There were many examples of formal purposeful play at Winston Grove, led by Gemma, but this kind of play did not offer up quite as much potential for free association among participants. Nonetheless, the informal moments found at Winston Grove – strikingly absent at Whittinghall – where care staff danced with residents, or joined in Daphne's wordplay, gave space to 'communicate a succession of ideas, thoughts, impulses, sensation' (p. 74) that were not necessarily linked but which helped to achieve a 'relaxation that belongs to trust and to acceptance... the resting state out of which a creative reaching-out can take place' (p. 74–75). Under the right circumstances, play became a space of possibility for the residents.

As Winnicott (1971) points out,

> It is in playing and only in playing that the individual child or adult is able to be creative and to use the whole personality, and it is only in being creative that the individual discovers the self.
>
> (p. 73)

When thinking of Daphne and Dorothy, we are not talking about the discovery of the self, but perhaps of recovering aspects of that self. It was clear that Daphne benefitted a great deal from moments of play. Many staff joined in with her 'Hey ho, it's off to work we go' or some other version. When she picked objects up in group activities, resignifying them, like a tambourine-turned-halo, staff were not critical but seemed to engage with her capacity for creating new symbols and meanings out of them. This was important to her, for her residual anxiety was of being seen as a 'silly sausage'. It was as if this release into play gave permission for people to encounter themselves in different states of mind, and for the staff to step out of their professional roles and engage on a different human level.

This seemed harder to achieve at Whittinghall, which appeared to package play up in clearly delineated timetabled spaces. During Dorothy's attendance at a flower-arranging activity the engagement with the co-ordinator was minimal. It felt staged, full of discomfort, as opposed to a potential space in which it were possible to re-experience the self, able to meet with whatever capacity for cognition. Following Winnicott's thinking (Winnicott, 2005, p. 75), even a lack of play in the clinical setting leads to a sense of hopelessness in the client, for she is unable to communicate nonsense. Whittinghall's approach to a time of play was to organise and timetable it, thereby denying the nonsense that, quite possibly, the residents needed to express.

Confusingly, time for play was available at Whittinghall but was not taken up because time was more commonly used for bureaucratic tasks and play (or rather break-time) for staff. To think of Armstrong (2005), play at Whittinghall punctuated interpersonal space by establishing conformity and routine as opposed to creating an interpersonal space in which mutual nonsense may have fostered connection. This communicated something about the implicit values woven into the fabric of organisational culture (managerialism foregrounded over relationships), and how national and local policy is perhaps interpreted at the level of the individual site.

By tapping into the way that Daphne played, much could be gleaned about her internal states. On one occasion Daphne played with a doll, inviting it to sit and look out on the lounge, as follows:

She takes the doll in her hands and looks into its eyes. 'Aren't you a special little one? Isn't he?' She looks quite the mother now. Daphne puts the doll back gently in a new position, its back resting on the back of the chair now. 'You can see the room better now,' she says. It's important to see things.

(Winston Grove)

With the use of this transitional object (Winnicott, 1953), Daphne seemed able to express her impulse for attachment and tenderness while also showing that she too was still capable of observing the world around her, like her doll. She was, in other words, connected and detached. As an object that was both me and not-me, her use of the doll was symbolic of a slow return to a mother, reconnecting with this earliest relationship while also sustaining a separate self. Daphne shifted into a maternal position and then back into herself. So here making time for play may help residents with dementia adapt to their shifting identities, in and out of dependence, and moments of continued relative independence.

Maude, introduced earlier in this chapter, also interacted with the soft toys in her bedroom as if they were transitional objects, all her teddies and soft toys. It was as if Maude drew on them to *be* in the world. Soft toys like Quack Quack and Winnie were used to create a potential space (Winnicott, 1960), a combination of inner and outer realities. Maude brought them to life, imbuing them with history and making them chat to one another as she and I were.

This potential space that had been created and discovered was one which allowed Maude to be comfortable in herself. She had the freedom to explore identities belonging to different periods of her life, through these soft toys and with me.

As Winnicott (1971) points out, 'The infant can employ a transitional object when the internal object is alive and real and good enough...' (p. 13). It was as if Maude's internal landscape allowed her to feel good about Winston Grove. She was not in a deeply melancholic state about being there, and was able to take in what she needed from the experience in order to sustain her in her dementia. Generally her view of Winston Grove was a benign one, resonant of a safe holding environment (Winnicott, 1960; 1962).

CONTAINER-CONTAINED: TIME TO THINK

The importance of finding time to think in both organisations was vital. Let us turn to Bion, for his work on containment provides a framework for the quality of thinking that is needed in dementia care. While Winnicott's focus was on a process that supported the development of an authentic sense of self, this was not Bion's focus. Bion highlights the importance of the mother-child relation in the formation of a thinking mind. Arguably, a mind able to think is also implicitly a mind of one's own, able to understand different feeling states and responses to situations. This leads to a form of getting to know, one surmises, oneself, and loosely relates to authenticity, but the emphasis is qualitatively different. Play doesn't necessarily lead to thinking, but being; containment leads to thought, thinking, and communication.

Play takes place externally, leading to creativity, to formations of culture, between people. Container-contained processes happen between people, and this process leads to the formation of mind, something structural, deeply internal. That said, this is too straightforward a reading, because both processes involve processes of projection, introjection, re-projection, and re-introjection. They are also processes or experiences we draw upon through the life course.

Klein's concept of projective identification was a germinating force behind Bion's container-contained. Bion (1962a) highlights intra-psychic processes more than the mother's physical and emotional responsiveness to the baby's signals, as Winnicott did.

The very mechanism of projective identification, though, at the basis of the container-contained process implies that there is an unconscious awareness in the infant of the mother being outside him in order to project something into her. Furthermore, the container-contained process can be a destructive one and, although in good circumstances it can lead to meaning-making and the development of a reflective mind, the projections from the baby are seen as an expulsion of intolerable fragments of experience, which are, in fantasy, sometimes violently pushed outwards.

Bion's (1962a) container-contained provides a detailed account of the way in which intra- and inter-psychic processes affect each party in the mother-infant dyad. This is particularly important for dementia care, where co-affecting moments take place between a professional carer and a person with dementia. Bion's explanation of containment and its relationship to a sense of continued existence also resonates:

> Normal development follows if the relationship between infant and breast permits the infant to project a feeling, say, that it is dying, into the mother and to reintroject it after its sojourn in the breast has made it tolerable to the infant psyche. If the projection is not accepted by the mother the infant feels that its feeling that it is dying is stripped of such meaning. It therefore reintrojects, not a fear of dying made tolerable, but a nameless dread.
>
> (Bion, 1962, p45)

Carers often receive such projections, and if they are unable to mobilise their alpha functioning (the thinking apparatus) in order to digest, to make sense of such projections, the projections are returned to the person with dementia in an unmanageable way. The mind is likely to continue to be in turmoil.

In a care home, feelings are often projected into the staff team. Similarly, feelings from the staff (i.e., feelings of vulnerability, hatred, love, and anxiety) are often projected into the residents. Although carers were able to contain the raw emotions of the residents at times, in both sites, the organisations themselves did not offer up spaces deliberately set up for thinking. Staff couldn't formally reflect upon what they might have become receptacles for, or about using the residents as projective objects for their own unwanted emotions. Thinking, in a Bionian sense, involves the ability to distinguish between conscious and unconscious thoughts, and leads to a capacity to be able to recognise one's motivations and one's role among others, to see oneself. Relatedly Bion's approach to containment, and the development of alpha-function, has been well used in the psychodynamics of organisational theory as evidence of the need for structured thinking spaces, as per the work of Armstrong (2005) and Lowe (2014).

If the opportunity for thinking is not part of care home culture, there are three possible consequences. The first is that communication might stay at an unconscious level, in a perpetual loop of forceful projections between staff and residents, which in turn would affect the capacity for either thinking or the holding on (for people with dementia) of mind. Secondly, as Bion points out, although projections might be more forceful, without a reflective alpha-function stance, the projections are 'denuded of the penumbra of meanings' (1962, p. 45); hence misunderstanding and misinterpretation would be common. Finally, thinking, in Bion's formulation, is closely linked with the capacity for communication and the articulation of truth-statements, which he argued was essential for harmonious group functioning. In Winston Grove, it was particularly evident that the need for the team to think together was vital.

We will remember that Diane made a link between the perception management had of her as doing harm, and her own vulnerability in the face of being thought of this way. Though we were unable to explore this link further, or to make it more conscious, our conversation offered the beginnings of a glimmer of containment. However, her need to speak about her experience pointed to a lack of time, at an organisational level, for staff to process sometimes unbearable feelings.

The conversation had enabled Diane to express the vulnerability that she registered in relation to the organisation and to her life. When Diane depicted Winston Grove as an inhumane place, likening it to 1970s London, in which she was excluded as a young black woman, the full force of her feeling of aloneness, rejection, came into view. We were able to touch upon this and do a little thinking about her vulnerability as a worker there. Diane implicitly addressed the way that projections moved around the organisation, from resident to staff member and back again, often unprocessed, left uncontained. A resident accuses Diane of abuse, and she in turn feels abused by management, the thinking about feelings of injury and of helplessness remains un-thought. People stay in pain, knowing at a deep level, but unable to formulate it clearly so others also know.

In terms of residents, the interview with Sue, the older woman from Wales who had recently moved into Winston Grove, had qualities of a therapeutic encounter in which a client's feelings might be projected into the therapist and thought about (Bion, 1962). Sue was able to process some of the raw feeling of loss she was experiencing when we talked about her experience.

Such a containing moment was unlikely to work for people with dementia if it were time-tabled or installed into a slot in the day. The containing moment needed to be in the here-and-now otherwise it would be lost. It made sense that, when containing encounters in the here-and-now were lacking, residents would return to past relationships, through which containing structures had been implanted. It was at these moments of non-containment and heightened anxiety, a mother (or occasionally a father) would be brought to life in residents' minds.

Time was a very interesting emergent category, particularly because it opened up avenues into thinking about the relational dynamics in both organisations, and what kinds of practices hindered or supported relationships. It highlighted omissions in policy; the reality of stretched workers endeavouring to relate to increasingly dependent others with minimal resources; and the strain of expectations of managerial efficiency.

Removing a coat from a resident who is anxious, and resettling them into a care home after a trip out demands the slowing down of time; walking with someone to a table when they are sturdy on their legs but wobbly of mind cannot be rushed. However, there are always momentary encounters which hold within them a meaningful experience of connection, perhaps a short spurt of time to play, to sing, to stroke a hand.

Equally, time for the 'super, super people', in Diane's words, is to be fought with and speeded up: a race against time, a competition between one's own efficiencies and the clock. Organisationally, time for reflection in both homes was hard to come by, and simultaneously hard to accept.

Elaine, the manager at Winston Grove, acknowledged the hardships that carers faced: '... staff do not have the time to spend with residents now... A lot of the time it is: get the tasks done and that's not the staff's fault.' Elaine seemed to understand how unrewarding this might be, identifying with the carers' position. She distanced herself from this kind of practice, implying that this development belonged to 'now', to the wider political environment, to her bosses' bosses in local and national arenas. Elaine imagined the punishing voice of senior management – 'get the tasks done' – to which she felt accountable, as did some members of staff. We have seen that without the time to think, to develop a containing organisational structure; without the time to work through anxieties through play, there is a tendency to become entrenched in widespread splitting as a defence against the emotional labour of the work and of the experience of having that work undervalued. It is essential that time be made available for different kinds of spaces, which allow for the sustaining of mind in both the workers and in people with dementia.

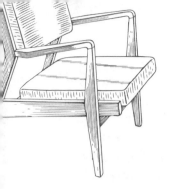

MOTHERS

ANDRE:	Andre? Nice name, Andre... Don't you think?
WOMAN:	It's a very nice name.
ANDRE:	My mother gave it to me, I imagine. Did you know her?
WOMAN:	Who?
ANDRE:	My mother.
WOMAN:	No
ANDRE:	She was so... She had very big eyes. It was... I can see her face now. I hope she'll come and see me sometimes. Mummy. Do you think? You were saying she might come occasionally for the weekend...
WOMAN:	Your daughter?

He's crushed by sudden grief.

ANDRE:	I want my mummy. I want her to come and fetch me. I want to go back home... I feel as if I'm losing all my leaves, one after another.

The Father, Florian Zeller (2015)

The maternal figure is a relevant one for care homes, for care work. Mother/s, although now dead, are brought to life seemingly for a variety of reasons; for emotional security (Miesen, 1993; 1999), yes, but also perhaps as a fantasised projective object in which to contain their difficult feelings. In a context where people are becoming increasingly dependent and are faced with death, we might imagine that some aspect of maternal love is yearned for, resonant of Kristeva's (1985) thinking.

Mothers are often called for by residents. This was the case particularly at Winston Grove. Care staff there made reference to their own mothers. Mothers figured in conversations with residents and staff at Winston Grove, and ideas about mother/s seemed to shape the way in which some residents sought to orientate themselves to their surroundings and to each other. Similarly, mothering informed how carers related to those they cared for.

At Whittinghall, Mother was notable by her very absence. Only one resident identified herself as a mother, albeit of a lost baby. The care staff talked about grandparents rather than mother/s, which seemed to relate to their youth and to the gap between the staff's generation and the residents'.

In his poem, 'The Old Fools', Philip Larkin (2003) imagined the minds of older people housing memories of those from lives gone by:

> *Perhaps, being old is having lighted rooms*
> *Inside your head, and people in them acting*
> *That is where they live*
> *Not here and now but when all happened once.*

> (p131)

People with dementia become increasingly dependent, and at this stage of life the maternal figure, a symbol of caring for dependent others, takes on a powerful presence in the erratically lighted rooms of fragmenting minds. This is evidenced in Browne & Shlosberg's (2012) study where participants often showed a mother fixation over and above a father one, a distinction not made by Miesen in his work on attachment-seeking behaviours in people with dementia (1993).

However, when carers feel overburdened by the emotional labour of the work, when there is simultaneously no organisational mother to support *them*, staff may avoid responding to the repetitive calls of the older people who cry out for their own mothers.

Winston Grove: Maternal care

Like the theme of time, the figure of the maternal was particularly alive at Winston Grove. Mothers with different qualities haunted both the culture, and the residents' minds. Residents sometimes called out for mothers – mothers who were dead and whose own children were soon to die.

This muddled, and muddling, merger of past and present lives and of being mothered, of having had mothers and, for some, of having been a mother to a child, was a striking reminder of who, and how, we are at our most fundamental. Always babies to mothers, always at some level having been connected to an-other: one that has given us a dwelling place within her body.

OUT OF TOUCH MOTHERS

Care staff or other residents also came to represent the particularity of mothers once known. Mothers were brought alive and feelings were sometimes projected into them – anxious mothers worried about disappearing children (the residents); containing mothers would soothe; lost mothers were searched for.

Mother was resurrected when Daphne was unwell, shivering in the activities room, upset that she wasn't being looked after – 'I don't know where my mother is. I don't know where she is at all' – or when she had returned to Winston Grove after a trip with her long-term partner, Benjamin. These scenes reveal how important the internalised maternal figure was for Daphne during anxious times, or when she felt ill-cared for.

> Daphne picks up her paintbrush and looks at it. She shivers all over again and puts it down on top of the palette of colours. 'Blue,' she says to herself.
>
> 'We are not being looked after,' says Daphne, visibly upset. 'They are all happy there.' She looks towards the end of the table towards Gemma. Daphne pulls her cardigan tight around her body and shivers again. She presses her hands together tightly and holds them together, her two thumbs interlocking.
>
> Daphne retreats into herself, a faraway look over her face.
>
> Daphne is still looking at the other members of the group. 'At least they like it,' she says, bursting into tears. 'I don't know where my mother is. I don't know where she is at all.' She coughs and then takes her left hand up to her throat.
>
> (Winston Grove)

Daphne clearly indicates that her mother would have provided care. Implied in Daphne's call for Mother is the perceived absence in that moment of good, attuned care. The activity continues and Daphne struggles on. Here Winston Grove is experienced as an out-of-touch mother, leaving Daphne alone, abandoned in the room.

ANXIOUS MOTHERS

Another day, Daphne had come back from a morning out with Benjamin. They had been to the cinema. On return, Daphne was confused: why was Benjamin no longer with her? She started to summon up her absent mother, imagining her worrying that Daphne was lost.

> *Daphne is standing in the main lounge, wearing a white blouse with grey flowers on. It has an open round neck. On top she wears a grey woollen cardigan. She is also wearing a mint-green pleated skirt and slippers. She has on her grey-rimmed glasses. 'I am worried that my mother'll be worrying about me, not being home,' says Daphne. She says nothing more. She starts walking out of the main lounge. As she walks down the short corridor, Daphne sees another resident – head down and making jerking movements with her hands that flop down to her side. This woman is leaving another lounge. Daphne stands aside. 'Well, when you see that she's here,' says Daphne, critically, implying this is not the right place for her.*
>
> (Winston Grove)

Daphne experiences herself as a lost girl, confused and concerned that no one – not even herself – knows where she is. Daphne communicates her lack of belonging and disconnection from the familiar, from home where Mother might be. Each week at Winston Grove brought new challenges for Daphne. By Christmas 2014, it seemed that Daphne was becoming less familiar with herself, and her context. She was moving away from herself as a woman in her eighties and remembering a younger self. As a result, whatever familiarity Winston Grove offered, it would never be as comforting as home, as Mother, as a childhood space and time. Through the imagined figure of Mother, Daphne seemed able to express her own anxious feelings about not being home. She retreats into being a child, expressing her feelings of dependence on another, who might help her achieve a more comfortable psychic state. At the end of this scene, sensing in Daphne a perturbing loneliness, I found myself sidling up to her, my body's movement itself saying, '*I am here with you.*'

COMFORTING MOTHERS

For Sue, whom we met in *Time*, asking questions about her life allowed her to open up enough to 'get back' in her mind to home with her mother and father. To remind the reader, Sue had recently moved into Winston

Grove, having been at hospital two weeks prior. There was a possibility that internally Sue was moving towards 'becoming-child' (Crociani-Windland, 2013, p. 347) – an ontological repetition that may facilitate, when noticed by others, comfort during periods of change and the working through of life's experiences. As Crociani-Windland (2013) notes so poignantly, 'We go back and we repeat, in order to go forward' (p. 348).

'When I was young going to school. So…' Sue pauses and takes a deep breath. 'Terrible ill, such nice people. And um I never forget it the goodness that you've done… have to get home to now.'

'Uh, everybody else lives there. Yes, but don't know how to get there anymore.' Sue is tearful and becomes silent. 'I'd like to go back.' Quiet again. 'Listen to the wind.' She hears this sound through the small opening in the window. She takes long breaths as she stares towards the trees outside.

'It's very very ill…' A pause. 'I'm very very surprised and thank you very much for helping me.' Sue laughs. 'I wouldn't know how to get back again. Yes, yes. It'll do cookery classes… and er… w… walking and things. And then we go tuh tuh tuh tuh.' Sue stamps her feet as if she is walking. 'That was a long time ago… Oh. It's very easy to find how to walk there now. Do you think so? It's terribly bad to forget things, isn't it? That's a long time ago now.'

It is as if Sue knows she is no longer a child, yet she has to allow herself to be one again. Speaking with her is painful.

'I just need to go home. It was where my mother and father… and go to chapel for things occasionally. I have to think how to get it over with. And then my mother is still alive so we can always have a chat. And then I can go back home… Yes. It's very very bad, isn't it when people go away?' Tears form in her eyes, and she lets out an 'ah'. 'Is there a bus ride… that is there a bus…? That there's a bus that we could get in and go half the way there or something like that. Speak to Mother and Father, and go to chapel again. Yes.'

(Winston Grove)

At a moment of great uncertainty, Sue summons up her parents and is compelled to return to them. Sue's parents represented a site of safety, familiarity. They would bring her back to a time when she was carefree, able to move without curtailment. The pain of loss for Sue is unbearable.

She has lost her home and her freedoms. A lost girl, unsure of how to get home. Listening, I feel impotent to help her in this quest. Yet the bearing witness to this deep sadness she is experiencing, arguably a function of the maternal or parental, is something Sue has been able to conjure up in me. I try to stay with what she is saying, allowing her to cry. There was a capacity at Winston Grove among the staff team to offer something akin to maternal containment (which Diane describes shortly). However, Sue evoked this responsiveness in me because she hadn't yet found it in her new surroundings. The reawakening memories, and vital attachments, held within them the painful experience of loss.

PRESENT MOTHERS

Daphne summoned up her mother, recognising her alive in other people, as a source of comfort as she walked around Winston Grove. Finding her mother within the care home seemed to suggest that sometimes Daphne felt at ease there.

Daphne follows the laminated corridor into a bright white kitchen area. The lights above dazzle, as if Daphne has emerged from the darkness of a tunnel. She looks out of the windows that give a full view onto another courtyard. Two chickens roam around on the paved area near their large coop. Both have the most ornate plumage. No ordinary chickens. A pigeon is looking back at Daphne through the window. Mutual curiosities, two-way mirrors, insides and outsides. 'He's taken a liking to you, you know,' Daphne turns to me and laughs.

Leaving the pigeon, she walks into the central lounge area. In the corner of the room, behind a dining table, a carer is taking out files from a cupboard. She places them on the table, opens one out and begins writing while another resident sleeps to the left of her. Spaces here are all-purpose: working, sleeping, eating.

'I will have to speak to him,' says Daphne, pointing at another female resident who is standing up, folding a napkin. This woman is hovering next to another lady, who is trying to talk to her. Daphne gets closer, seeking proximity. She says hello but there is no reply. Daphne walks away to the back of the room and sits down. She does not seem offended. Daphne watches the resident with the napkin in her hand. 'My mum,' says Daphne. You can't help but notice the gentle expression on Daphne's face as she recognises her mum in this resident. Her lips turn ever so slightly

into a smile, eyes softening. 'It's good, I suppose, really, at least she gets to know lots of new people now. It can't be bad.'

(Winston Grove)

Here Daphne revived a mother who was relaxed, settling in. The function of Daphne's shadowy mother was often to be a mirror to her own experience. Daphne was so comfortable in this scene that she was able to take notice of her environment and the people in it, in much the same way that I spent my time noticing her, taking her in. There was, it seemed, a ripple effect of noticing which was mirror-like in itself.

For the staff team, too, the maternal figure was sometimes able to provide comfort.

Mother at work

This is Chaya, a carer at Winston Grove, who immediately summoned up the maternal in her work.

REPARATION

Chaya has worked at Winston Grove for over eight years. She wears her hair tied back. She is presentable, smiling a great deal, with her eyes. Her voice is gentle, she is keen to talk. A circle of chairs is in the middle of the room in which we talk, following an exercise session. Overhead are photocopied fish, some exotic, some recognisable, painted in wild colours by the residents.

'I enjoy myself because being with the people living with experience of dementia, uh, talking to them and, you know, getting to know them and looking after them after, you know them, I feel it's very... I am very happy about it, I am interested and I'm mostly happy because my mum she lived with the experience of dementia and at that time I did not know what was dementia, I was not trained and or anything like that and my mum passed away and I came here and after I, you know...' Chaya stops. 'After I was trained and got so much of knowledge about it I really, really enjoyed working with them and I feel sorry that I didn't have that experience when Mum was alive, um, yeh... because, you know, I feel in these people, I see my mum. I mean, I know from up above she must be thinking okay, you know like I really enjoy what I'm doing.'

'My mum died of infection, like now I know like when they have any kind of, that kind of moments like, you know like they're not themselves

like it's a UTI. My mum had a lot of moments like that and I not know, nobody told me. Was kind of overlooked and she had very very bad... and that's how she passed away. I think if I had have known this I think she would be still alive.'

Chaya explains what she gets from doing the work, what she gets from the residents.

'... well, the happiness and they know they are understood, you know, and they are happy like.' A resident walks in quietly then leaves. 'Like him [she says talking about the man who has just come and gone], I think two years back he was sitting in the lounge and that day it was a very hectic day and I was doing medication and the people were running around and some was moving around the table and some was crying. In the middle of medication all these things happening so it was very very challenging that particular evening and he was sitting in own corner of the lounge and I was running about giving medication and coming back. I came into the lounge and he says, "Here she comes, the light of my life."' She smiles, laughs. 'It was so, so nice. You know, you know all that tension it just went away... It was so nice... So many people, so many of them... there's examples from so many residents. It gives you so much of happiness. Another... Jane was like sitting at the table and the night staff were telling her it was time to go to bed, the night staff were telling her... and as soon as she saw me she was just holding her hands like that [opened out, palms upwards]... "If there was an angel on this earth that's you."'

Chaya reflects on her mother, on what she knows now.

'I am sad that I didn't have that knowledge when I was looking after my mum, I'm very sad about that but I feel her presence always there and you know each stage of her life I can see in these residents, each stage of their life... It's nice, I love working with them, it's... but if you don't understand them, if I didn't have the training it'd be difficult... like with Mum, like when she had those anxious moments and she was walking around and I used to get, get actually, sometimes I'd get a little bit angry, I'd say, "Mum I just told you... now please sit down." I did not know, I did not know that they had anxious moments and I did not know how to approach and Mum was... when I was looking after Mum but now I've got knowledge. You know that strength... she's given me that strength. As soon as I entered a home for work I could feel my mum's presence and that's how I got stuck into it.'

(Winston Grove)

Chaya's work is unequivocally related to maternal function and practice. It is as if Chaya mobilises not just memories of her mother but an internal mother with whom she is in identification.

For Chaya, being at Winston Grove is an act of reparation expressed through her choice of work (Klein, 1952). She is doing for the residents what she felt unable to do for her mum. Daily life at Winston Grove allows her to reconnect with her absent yet ever-present mother. Chaya explains that she recognises the stages of her mother's life in the residents. Resonant of Ettinger's (2006) work on the matrixial field, we see how Chaya interacts with the residents as individuals partially through the lens of this internalised mother with dementia. Chaya casts herself both in the position of a good-enough carer to the residents yet one who came up short in relation to her own mother.

MATERNAL FAILINGS

Different qualities of the maternal – angry, thoughtful, failing, anxious mothers– also emerged in the work. Here Elaine, the manager of Winston Grove, reflects upon a situation in which she feels responsible for failing her team.

> Elaine is an efficient woman, well dressed and energetic. She laughs a lot and often gets her hands dirty. She is quick and to the point, cautious about what she says.
>
> 'In fairness no. They don't [the staff]… they don't complain. Um and sometimes I think they should have done especially I know when Roger (a former assistant manager) left and things were quite heavy but because I was short-staffed office-wise they didn't want to be coming to me saying look we need… 'cos they told the Inspector because it was her that told me and I said well look that's not fair if they do have a genuine issue then they should bring it to my attention so I can do something about it. It was only when I was… I put the float back in that… because staff hadn't been coming to me saying look we need extra help at this time of the morning or that time of the evening… they hadn't been coming and saying it whereas if I had I could have done something about it sooner.'
>
> 'When I was made aware of it I put a shift back in… it was needed.'
>
> Elaine explains that the staff did not come to her, but mentioned the difficulties to the Inspector. She makes sense of this by imagining a team of staff, protecting her.

'... they were trying to be nice in a way but they weren't helping themselves. You know, "she's got enough stress going on without adding to it..." They... would have been better if they'd just come along and said "look we're really struggling here now we need to do something about it," and it would have been done.'

(Winston Grove)

Elaine described a situation in which the Care Quality Commission Inspector had made an unannounced visit, at a time when there were many staff shortages and the team felt under pressure. Instead of asking Elaine for the reintroduction of a helping carer, who would move between groups, filling in gaps, some members of staff spoke to the Inspector. Common to leader/follower relations, Elaine imagines that the staff team were protecting her, unwilling to make further demands on her directly. Relations to authority figures are often tinged with feelings, partly conscious, that come from earlier child-parent relations. Although Elaine does not refer to these relations directly, they might have been present in some degree in the way the staff saw her and how she saw them. Elaine considered herself a robust enough figure to have heard their concerns, but at that time the staff team felt otherwise. In this instance, Elaine was unable to contain the anxieties and respond to the needs of the team yet she does not want to dwell on this situation – possibly because there are further interpretations less benign that she does not want to entertain.

MATERNAL MEANING-MAKER

In contrast, Diane, who talked about racism in the UK, provides an eloquent account of meaning-making involved in day-to-day care work, demonstrating how important the consciously reflective mind of a carer can be in supporting feelings of integration in residents with dementia. Here she is able to show a very different side to Winston Grove to the one she described earlier. The representation of the organisation in her mind is now imbued with a capacity for careful attunement.

Diane spoke this way.

'I always think like that. This could be Mum or Dad at ninety-four. It's silly and it's soppy and it's uneconomical but I always think like that. It doesn't tick any of the right boxes but if I didn't do it that way I couldn't *come to work. I'd have no motivation to even come in the door, there'd be nothing in it for me. It's okay earning a wage packet, but if your heart is not in it you don't want it. Don't want it.' Diane sobs. 'When my heart's no longer in it I can't do it.'*

'You have to like people and you have to understand people and they're here because they need care. They need support, they're pretty vulnerable. Sometimes they can't express themselves, sometimes they forget, they might start a sentence and then forget it. You have got to fill in the blank spaces and do what you have to do.'

(Winston Grove)

The spectre of the maternal (or paternal) figure is both unsettling in the work, yet helpful. Conjuring up her parents moves Diane – it is arguably at the heart of the work for her – and brings certain emotional realities into the frame. All sorts of questions might arise: how will I bear the undeveloping of my parents? How did I treat them? Was I a good or bad child? What is interesting in this construction is that carers might position themselves as children in relation to imagined parents, who are nonetheless dependent. It is a reversal of the original parent-infant dynamic.

Yet Diane also sees herself as a mothering figure, suggesting that she is sometimes able to provide a containing function, in a Bionian sense, when she takes in some of the confused parts of the residents and attempts to re-present them in meaningful ways. When we think of the organisation-in-the-mind, it seems that the brutal organisation Diane had described sometimes had a capacity for empathy. Diane understands that dementia involves the experiencing of holes, spaces, gaps that unsettle being. Part of her role is to make sense of the holes, to fill them with meaning. Implicitly she has to keep the thread-like moments of being alive in her mind so that a social-emotional death does not ensue. Diane conceives of a carer's role as one that sustains psychic continuity. The carer, like the mother, is involved in an interactive collaboration which, through being present to associations and omissions, helps someone to be known. Maternal functions, such as this one, act in counterpoint to efficiency and proceduralism. Indeed, as we shall see from Celia's discussion of being interrupted, sometimes delaying the task in hand (inefficiency) allowed care workers to bridge the gap between them and the residents, to make meaning as part of a co-constructive process.

MATERNAL INTERRUPTIONS

Celia from Winston Grove, whom we met in *Time*, had some interesting and paradoxical thoughts on interruptions in her care practice.

'... dementia care should be personal centred... It should be about continuity but I find that we don't have that at the minute because we don't have the sort of staffing, um, you can find yourself working with new people on a regular basis. Take this past couple of days, Saturday, Sunday, Monday, three different people, today and yesterday I'm working with this guy I worked with yesterday and today where is the continuity there? You know, it throws a lot back on you as permanent staff because you have to stop to give an induction to this person, telling them about the residents and some residents don't like new unfamiliar faces and voices so it means more is put back on you, the permanent care staff, 'cos you now have to go to do M [a male resident].'

'Because if he doesn't know you and you don't know how to deal with him because he doesn't express, "Oh, I'm hungry". It's like we determine whether he's had something, so before we even go to do personal care... you offer him a drink or a banana or something then he's much calmer for you to deal with him. People who don't know him say, "Oh he's lashing out, he's this, he's that," so for me that's where the continuity is important. You need to have the staff that know the sort of user... you have different individuals to care for and everybody living with dementia is an individual and presents different challenges and if they don't know them then that's where we stuck... The, the continuity of staff and yes they say personal-centred care but for me it's not happening.'

(Winston Grove)

For Celia, the staff team were experiencing permanent and negative interruptions in the form of regular temporary workers coming in to fill spaces. This related to austerity measures within social care. These fill-in roles were experienced as a 'seemingly endless series of micro-blows' (Baraitser, 2006, p. 68) to good, coherent care. Care staff felt more under pressure, taking on the dual role of caring and training on the job.

However, there was a paradox at the heart of Celia's discussion on interruption. In relation to the temporary worker, interruption severs understanding. When Celia allows herself to be interrupted personally by a resident, then something more positive is brought to light, as follows:

'It can be, it can be. It can be very frustrating but as for me you have to find the time to do the one-to-one and you can't rush these people because like D [a male resident] he has his good days and his bad days. One day he'll try to explain carefully what he wants to say and one day he was walking in the garden, I'll give you an example... He wanted me to go in the garden and he said, "Come, come," and I said, "D I can't I have got to give out medication," and he said, "Come come." So I ended up having to put away the medication and I had to say to Alan [the caretaker], "Do not ignore them." We cannot, and D took me outside and where was he carrying me, taking me to the outhouse where the pads were stored. Alan and I went there early and we were putting the pads in and, knowing we'd come back, we left the door open so that's what D was calling to show me that the door was open, that the breeze had opened the door.'

'The pad door was open and I had a list with all of these pads so I was putting it away and I pushed in the door but no I didn't lock it. Well D saw it wide open so he came to get me you know so. But it's like he cannot express himself so you have to stop, listen, engage, and just go with him and he's only one of many. Oh he can't get it out and when he can't get it out he will let out one or two swear words because he cannot verbally express what he wants to tell you. This needs time. This needs time. You cannot rush care you cannot compromise care. You have to find out what they are trying to show you...'

(Winston Grove)

Resonant of Baraitser's (2009) work on mothering and interruption, Celia notes a moment when she is called upon to confront an ethical dilemma and perhaps a series of powerful feelings in herself – frustration, hopelessness – in doing so. Does she continue to give medication or does she follow D? Speaking of the way such breaches characterise mother-child relating, Baraitser (2009) writes of the '...tears, puncturings to the mother's durational experiences' (p. 68) which bring her time after time 'into the realm of the immediate... the here and now of the child or infant's demand' (p. 68). As we have seen in some of the observations (e.g., Suki's calls for the toilet, Dorothy's 'Wendy, Wendy, Wendy'), when residents cry out and interrupt the continuity of one task or another, that cry serves the purpose of eliciting care from the care worker. Here, D demands a caring, concerned response yet he also offers care simultaneously.

Celia allows herself to be interrupted on this occasion, her activity punctured. Paradoxically this rupture leads to a deeper connection with D, with them both now effectively working together, recognising (Benjamin, 2006) one another. The interruption itself acts as a catalyst for reflection, perhaps giving Celia greater access to her own complex subjectivity and to D's. This process was possible when the grip of linear clock time was loosened, where one person's time frame, sense of personal continuity, could make room for another's.

Celia's thinking about interruption showed it wasn't just 'depleting but generative' (Baraitser, 2009, p. 69). There was some sense here that organisationally Winston Grove could hold together, and think about, paradoxical experiences and modes of being that were both dislocating and constructive.

Whittinghall: Maternal care

The kind of meaning-making Diane describes, and Celia's learning from interruption, seemed unavailable at Whittinghall. Dorothy's repetitions were understood only as a symptom of her dementia, the underlying significance never investigated. The same was true of Evie who called out 'Johnny' in a haunting voice. To become involved in a process of meaning-making with another person, some curiosity (Klein, 1930) is vital. Whittinghall often seemed uninterested in and impermeable to the affective experience of its residents and thus the organisation was not always able to produce a sense of going-on-being in the older people. Investigating Dorothy's and Evie's repetitions may have offered up more generative possibilities, allowing them to find the lost object/s they called for before finally letting go. Given that the maternal was central to learning and meaning-making at Winston Grove, it is probably unsurprising that their relative absence from Whittinghall was accompanied by an absence of mothers.

ABSENT MOTHERS

In Whittinghall, the maternal figure barely featured in the minds of residents. Dorothy never cried out for her mother, and talked about her own daughter only once. The daughter, in turn, was said to visit rarely. It was during the penultimate observation that Dorothy seemed to create a link between her daughter and home, as if her mothering experience reminded her of a time which provided comfort. As Matthew Desmond (2016) tells us in his painfully human depiction of eviction in Milwaukee, 'Home is the centre of life… We say that at home we can "be ourselves." Everywhere else, we are someone else. At home, we remove our masks… The home is the well-spring of personhood. In languages spoken all over the world, the word for "home" encompasses not just shelter but warmth, safety, family – the womb. The ancient hieroglyph for "home" was often used in place of "mother".' (p. 293)

In the following vignette, time at Whittinghall was beginning to come to an end:

> *Evie is missing still. But so is Dorothy. Her absence is striking, dislocating.*
>
> *It is good to see Dorothy sitting with a group of residents and an activities co-ordinator, in her burgundy tunic. Many residents are sitting in wheelchairs. She is seated next to a woman with glasses on. Dorothy's chin is resting on her hands, her forehead and face down. Her eyes are slightly closed. Dorothy asks if it's time to go home. She asks Nancy about 'Fiona' and where she is. Fiona is Dorothy's adopted daughter but she is not coming today. Dorothy puts her head down again, saddened. She wants to go home.*
>
> *Nancy asks Dorothy if she has enjoyed herself; she says she doesn't know. Nancy brings the rose that Dorothy has placed in a vase closer to her, and says that it's a beautiful colour – it is yellow.*
>
> *The activities co-ordinator jokingly says that Nancy is disturbing her. 'I'd like to know how to get back home,' Dorothy looks towards the window. 'I don't know what I am supposed to be doing here. I don't know,' she says. She looks out of the window and notices it is raining again. 'I don't know what to do, I think it is time for home.'*
>
> …
>
> *Dorothy seems to fall asleep, her breathing heavier. Perhaps, asleep, she'll somehow find home.*
>
> (Whittinghall)

MEMORIES OF THE BABY

Another of the infrequent references to mothers at Whittinghall was in conversation with Ellen, a gentle but worried resident. Ellen presented herself as a mother and yet she seemed representative of a baby in the grip of a dreadful fragmentation, dependent and scared. It was as if she were the baby without a responsive mother, an image that married up with time spent in the home.

There were several plants and photos on a window-ledge in Ellen's room. Dressed in dark browns, with wispy hair falling in front of her face, Ellen struggled to get her bearings. This played out in her trying to decide which shoes to wear. Ellen's dementia may have impaired her sense of body schema. At one point Ellen takes my foot as though it is her own, a phantom body-part, symbolic of her disconnection with the immediate environment. So hard to witness, had Ellen become a series of part-objects to herself?

'And the fellow that's the [mumbles] house was housing up here, was very airy. It was awful. A little girl got there. Think it was the daughter's child. They were well I think, but I was quite glad to be able to try with mine. But… I don't… it's a crazy world. I don't know where I am, how I am… I feel quite deaf today. Usually I can hear okay but this… I don't know what I was doing today and when and why. The look in his eyes and we are going to do this this and this. I didn't take anything home. It was very strange. All the way to go. Thought where is my baby…? Have I left her behind? He's not very old. I can't remember. Things aren't working well with me. I can't seem to keep top of… I don't know what mistakes pop and… those aren't mine.'

Ellen picks up her shoe, taking one of her slippers off and trying on another shoe.

'You won't believe it, there's two. What's that one doing there? Doesn't quite like but it's not bed. Bright like.' *Ellen laughs out loud.* 'I don't know that I like the bright red ones really. Bother… Oh it goes with those. Yes it does. That's that. Oh it changes it's… Oh what's this one doing? Oh. I'm going crackers.'

(Whittinghall)

Ellen herself is the mother who has lost her own baby. Simultaneously, the lost baby is representative of Ellen. She is both mother and baby, someone losing and someone lost. It seemed important to stay with her in her confusion. She was continually flicking the hair out of her eyes, changing one shoe for the other, her laughter the only way of making it bearable. Her shoes, like the sparse room and her slippery words, felt as though they didn't belong to her. Ellen's fragmentation was powerful, and it didn't seem coincidental that she was the only resident who referred to a baby per se, reminding us perhaps of Winnicott's (1960) infant gripped with the fear of disintegration.

THE ABSENT ORGANISATIONAL MOTHER

The image of Ellen as a baby fragmenting in the absence of a responsive mother echoed something of the emotional quality of Whittinghall, namely as somewhere in which an overarching organisational mother was absent. This absence was particularly felt in relation to the psychic confusions and disintegration of the residents and was manifest in the staff's care practice.

The staff could be impenetrable, which surely caused further panic and dislocation in the residents, in their experience of dementia.

> 'Wendy, Wendy, Wendy,' shouts Dorothy. Louder, louder, louder. She raises her hand into the air and makes that bird-like beak shape with her hand. 'What am I doing, doing, doing?' she says. Nancy doesn't answer nor does the other carer. Dorothy shakes her head and puts her face in her hands. 'Don't know what I'm doing, doing, doing.' Nancy is busy filling in forms, not noticing what Dorothy is saying.
>
> (Whittinghall)

In what follows, a male carer allows himself to be interrupted by one resident, abandoning another in the process. You wonder, given the lack of eye contact, if both residents are seen as tasks to be completed. Certainly, there is no sense here of responsive maternal care.

> The male carer doesn't make eye contact with the man but starts following him to where he needs to go, leaving Evie in the chair in the middle of the corridor. Abandoned. She says nothing, her feet dangling from the chair. 'Don't like the look of that,' says Dorothy, noticing Evie's predicament. She shakes her head. The phone starts going again but no one answers.
>
> (Whittinghall)

There were many examples of the absent mother at Whittinghall. Here, if Mother is present, we find mothering of a noticeably distant, uninterested kind.

He (the waiting staff) hands the woman next to Dorothy a Hobnob. He gives the lady next to her another biscuit. The man opposite Dorothy is sitting in a wheelchair; his body looks stiff and his arms are bent in front of him. A debilitating long-term condition perhaps. The man in the waiter's costume walks past him, doesn't hand him a biscuit. The man uncomfortably twists his body round looking at the biscuit tray. He looks confused but says nothing. The waiter puts the tray in front of a man next to the man in the wheelchair, and holds the tray still for some minutes. The activities co-ordinator reaches over the man and takes a piece of cake for herself. Begins eating it.

The man in the wheelchair with the contorted body is looking ahead now, silent but sad. After some minutes, the activities co-ordinator walks around to him with a piece of soft cake in a napkin. She takes a tiny amount of cake between her finger and thumb. 'You are my darling,' she says. She holds the morsel towards his mouth. He looks at it with his eyes narrowing, and then he takes it with his mouth. She continues to feed him like this, without speaking, chewing her own piece of cake and looking ahead at the rain out of the window as she does so. It is a picture you see in cafes when mums give bottles to their babies while staring at their phones, an image of disengaged giving.

(Whittinghall)

The man in the wheelchair is forgotten. He says nothing but his eyes looked pained. What made the disconnected mode of relating so hard to bear was the fact that this man was so physically incapable of helping himself. Although the activities co-ordinator began with some impulse of generous mothering, the feeding of the cake, usually a good point of contact when Nancy fed Dorothy, gradually became something task-focused and absent of feeling, the initial generosity hard to sustain.

Family constellations: the staff team

If staff care practices frequently suggested the absence of an overarching organisational mother, it is probably unsurprising that, in contrast to Winston Grove, mothers were almost never mentioned in staff interviews. Grandparents were more commonly discussed, however, possibly because the care team was made up of younger workers. Generationally this kind of conceptualisation made sense. Nancy spoke of being treated as a grandchild and even – and this felt uncomfortable to hear – admitted that sometimes the staff called certain residents granddad or grandma. Although these comments were presented as cheerful and fond, these kind of references were too casual, blithe: real identities overshadowed by distanced make-believe ones.

> *Prashid, a male carer, speaks for a few minutes. There is loud classical music playing in the background. All the tables are dressed for lunch with wine glasses and napkins. Prashid seems reluctant to talk, tentative about revealing too much.*
>
> 'Well I like working here because it's a bit different job than I did before. Personally I have changed so many things in my life and this job it has impacted. Working with elderly people it's like … you know, my culture… the culture I come from we care more about elderly people so normally we don't have care homes… back home… we look after our grandparents and our relatives. So when I first started this job I felt like I'm back into my culture and working like. I felt it like that. I built up my patience and communicating so lots of things have improved… we don't have care homes there… facilities-wise we are very much backwards but here we have loads of facilities but I'm not very familiar with the culture… Looking at the facilities here it's very good… I used to look after my grandparents but not really in a working environment. Here it's like a job but it's like a home as well.'
>
> (Whittinghall)

Prashid speaks indirectly about his grandparents. This link to people in his life reminds him of his home country. He resignifies Huntside unit from work to home. In fact, this tendency to talk about work in terms of 'family' or 'home' was one of the most striking things about Whittinghall. However, the family was one in which the mother and, for that matter, the father, were not present. The greatest connections were among members of the staff team themselves: there were photographs by the nurses' station of staff Christmas parties; surprising moments of intimate touch between individual staff members; and staff were often seen going off on breaks in groups. If the organisation-in-the-mind for members of the staff team took on a family-like quality, it was as a constellation of siblings where grandparents featured in the distance and parents were wholly absent.

Understanding mother/s

The absence of the maternal figure in Whittinghall was pronounced. Residents did not cry out for mothers of any sort and staff did not reference their own parents. To return to the organisational picture, we might imagine that Mother here had delegated her role. The children are doing the care while she remains aloof and out of reach.

Mothers imbued with different qualities were present in Winston Grove. They were often summoned up by residents, as if feelings belonging to them could usefully be projected onto fantasised figures from the past. This mechanism seemed to make way for the expression of a vast array of feelings that belonged to the residents, but which ended up being located in 'mother'. This might have meant that different aspects of maternal care (good, bad, and in-between) were in fact present at Winston Grove.

As the reader will have seen, mother/s often appeared at Winston Grove. Daphne regularly made sightings of her mother, embodied in different residents. It was noticeable that the figure of the mother she evoked took on certain affective qualities. It was as if these maternal figures became containers for Daphne's own unwanted anxieties. When Daphne felt lost or alone, she would imagine her mother worrying about her well-being or safety. It is possible that Daphne found this projection into an imagined or symbolic realm a helpful way of communicating her own uncertain state. There were also times when Daphne projected into a surrogate mother figure (usually a resident) a feeling of greater ease, communicating something about her own immediate experience of comfort.

The way that Daphne mobilised an internal mother was something repeated by many residents, often when they felt homeless or worried. These maternal figures (internal hauntings and memories) were brought back to life quite possibly in order to anchor the residents. Sometimes mothers were located in care workers; sometimes in residents. Staff also imagined in the residents their own mothers. It was clear that at Winston Grove, there was a role for the maternal.

In contrast, at Whittinghall, Dorothy did not call upon her mother. Similarly, staff members did not refer to mother/s. A possible conclusion was that the organisational function of mothering was thin on the ground. It could be argued that the metaphorical caring mother had delegated her role, leaving it in the hands of paid staff.

At Winston Grove, where mother/s were mentioned, there was seemingly a distinct difference in the way that staff and residents made use of the mother figure. The residents seemed to mobilise an internal mother, as a source of holding and of containment. For the staff – particularly in Chaya – there were identifications with an internal mother who was possibly part deprived of her care, which was offered to the residents in an act of reparation.

I want to say more about Chaya's account, as it was a powerful evocation of mother/s in the work, and the act of reparation that might have motivated, in part, many to become carers.

MOTHERS: GUILT AND REPARATION

Chaya was striking because her reasons for working at Winston Grove were closely tied to memories of her mother, of looking after her. Chaya had been her mother's primary carer when she succumbed to dementia, though Chaya had at the time been unaware of the diagnosis and of what this meant. Chaya acknowledged feeling out of her depth and frustrated with her mother, unclear why her behaviour was changing. Chaya had been ashamed of this, but once trained she recognised behaviours in the residents she had seen in her own mother. For her, getting a job at Winston Grove had, in a sense, allowed her to go home to Mother. Chaya's words read like an ode to the human capacity, and need, for reparation. She made references to angels. Listening to Chaya, you imagined Winston Grove to be a site of perfect care, of the Virgin Mary. At times, unthinkingly idealised, and among more critical accounts (Diane's, for example) Chaya's account was strikingly optimistic. Chaya had felt guilt, we might surmise, for having damaged the maternal object. Working as a carer helped to make the damage better through her continual exemplary care towards others.

In order to understand the reparative compunction as a guiding principle of care and welfare work, it might be useful to turn to those working in the Kleinian tradition. As Froggett (2010) notes,

At first sight, then, Klein's work seems unpromising as a basis for models of welfare which seem to require a degree of optimism regarding our ability to care for one another... it is difficult to find its justification in a view of the mind that identifies a persistent potential for destruction: in which split 'paranoid-schizoid' states are part of normal functioning; in which the propensity for gratitude and love is described in terms of the achievement of a 'depressive position'... Yet despite, or perhaps because of, the fact that we are condemned to an ongoing struggle between our love and our hate, there is in Klein an account of love in which it is possible to discover not only our capacity for destruction but also our ability to make good the damage that we do. It is the reparative impulse born of guilt and gratitude that forms the basis of ethical life. This lends itself to an understanding of compassion – love directed to recognition of and care for the other.

(p. 36)

As we know, it is within the infant-mother relationship that these first acts of psychic reparation take place. Let us go directly to Klein:

The anxiety relating to the internalised mother who is felt to be injured, suffering, in danger of being annihilated or already annihilated and lost for ever, leads to a stronger identification with the injured object. This identification reinforces both the drive to make reparation and the ego's attempts to inhibit aggressive impulses... This tendency, as we have seen earlier, is inextricably linked with feelings of guilt. When the infant feels that his destructive impulses and phantasies are directed against the complete person of his loved object, guilt arises in full strength and, together with it, the over-riding urge to repair, preserve or revive the loved injured object. These emotions in my view amount to states of mourning, and the defences operating to attempts on the part of the ego to overcome mourning... The reparative tendency too, first employed in an omnipotent way, becomes an important defence. The infant's feelings might be described as follows: 'My mother is disappearing, she may never return, she is suffering, she is dead. No, this can't be, for I can revive her.'

(pp. 74–5)

Chaya's interview showed that there was a capacity, from an organisational perspective, of facing loss from a depressive position. Despite the overall idealisation of the work, Chaya is able to recognise both the love for her mother and the frustrations, anger, she experienced towards her. In facing this ambivalence, she restores her mother as a whole object, and her own ego, able to experience and re-experience her feelings of loss.

For others at Winston Grove, the reviving of mothers was perhaps representative of a strand of institutional defence, which guarded against mourning all those loved objects who perhaps no longer visited or were no longer alive. Though the residents and staff were not infants it is possible that working in a place where losses were so pervasive meant that the resurrection of mothers also related to ongoing omnipotent fantasies of keeping people alive – this does seem to fit with Winston Grove's overall tendency to deny the fear of death.

HOLDING

A further function of the mother figure was – particularly for some of the residents – the provision of some kind of holding, particularly in times of difficulty and distress. This enabled residents to go on being both in a temporal and spatial sense. As Winnicott (1960) notes,

> The term 'holding' is used here to denote not only the actual physical holding of the infant, but also the total environmental provision prior to the concept of living with. In other words, it refers to a three-dimensional or space relationship with time gradually added. This overlaps with, but is initiated prior to, instinctual experiences that in time would determine object relationships. It includes the management of experiences that are inherent in existence, such as the completion (and therefore the non-completion) of processes, processes which from the outside may seem to be purely physiological but which belong to infant psychology and take place in a complex psychological field, determined by the awareness and the empathy of the mother.
>
> (p. 589)

As we saw from Ellen's story on page 157, holding might have offered her a sense of temporal continuity in counterpoint to the experience of psychic and physical fragmentation.

Ogden (1986), referring to Winnicott's work, states:

> If we view holding as dominant among the functions of the mother in the earliest stage of development, and weaning as the dominant function in the period of the transitional phenomenon, in the depressive position the critical task of the mother can be conceived of as surviving over time.
>
> (p. 191)

Holding, offered to the pre-verbal infant by its mother, supports the continued development of a child's emotional and psychic reality. The baby's survival over time is in a sense related to the mother's survival over time. I want to focus on holding because, although containing mothers were also, and importantly, brought to life, containment, in a Bionian sense, does not operate in this distinctly temporal mode. For Ellen, it is her un-development that is striking. Her words seem out of reach, and you might have thought that she was returning to a set of experiences which were less about sustaining the structure of a thinking mind (Bion, 1962), and more about finding a way to support a sense of ongoing-ness.

Holding is, in Winnicott's view, a function of the mother or primary carer. It includes both bodily – via handling – and emotional care to support ego integration. Although 'holding' can be done by anyone (indeed it can be done through institutional arrangements), in a culture where mothers do most of the close caring for and nurturing of infants, holding is inevitably imbued with maternal associations.

I will say a little more about Ellen because I wondered if my sitting with her un-ravelling seemed to offer something of the quality of a brief holding experience. We might imagine that the baby is the prototypical subject of care, dependency, and responsibility. In Whittinghall, the holding environment was shaky. Rather than carers making careful attempts to reflect the residents' emotional states or to adapt to their needs, the staff seemed to erect a boundary between them and the residents that foreclosed empathic response. This was seen in the staff congregating around the nurses' station, impervious to Dorothy's cries; the need for staff to use their water bottles (not the home's glasses, used by the residents); the talk of holidays, breaks; and the photos of staff nights' out dotted around the station.

This was very much in contrast to the purpose of holding that Winnicott envisages where an infant's being is sustained, owing to the thoughtful responsiveness of the mother, the bedrock of 'human reliability' (Winnicott, 1987). Of course, residents in a care home are not infants, but I did wonder whether the intense levels of dependency experienced by some people with dementia, like Ellen, made one-to-one highly responsive care essential, that a holding response, of the sort Winnicott describes, was an appropriate one. Ellen even misrecognised my foot for her own, symbolising perhaps a powerful need for connection and imagined unity. Very early on, I understood intuitively that questioning

Ellen was unlikely to be helpful to her. Instead, I made myself available to her need to go over and repeat a part of herself, the internal child, which seemed to help her to manage the intensity of her distress. This intense distress is apparent, for instance, in the moment when she said 'I go total blank... most of the pieces aren't here...'

If we think of Evie, too, who occasionally sat in the corridor next to Dorothy, there was an instance where Amy, the home manager, insisted that she keep trying to stand up with her walker. There was not much sympathy shown for the frail body that might have wanted to be held in place. In the absence of instances of maternal holding at Whittinghall, it was tempting to consider the organisation as one that either proactively valued standing on one's own feet – independence – over a supportive holding (interdependence); or one that denied the existence of need. Arguably the two were related but not entirely the same. That said, there were also equivalent instances at Winston Grove – take the lady with impaired sight who was marched, precariously dancing, to a lunch table; and Suki's desperate cries to be toileted, which went ignored.

A holding environment, then, is about the mother's early good enough adaptability to the infant's needs, both the way the baby is 'held in the mother's mind as well as in her arms' (Phillips, 2007, p. 30). This process can only be done well on the basis of the mother's imaginative elaboration of the infant's states, feeding into the structure of the infant's psychological matrix. In other words, through her capacity to translate the cries, a communication, Mother becomes mirror-like in her responsiveness, thus creating within the infant the sense of reliability and security which set the foundations for ongoing ego strength.

For Winnicott (1960), a good holding environment for the infant is tied up with the move from dependence to relative dependence and on to further independence, which he argues can only be successfully achieved if the child is able to draw on memories of dependable maternal care which thus offers a sense of confidence in the environment. Winnicott's notion of holding is, from a maternal-infant care perspective, a generally positive experience, an almost sensuous experience for the infant, a building block towards a sense of internal safety.

It is quite possible, in dementia care, that the person with dementia feels more at ease and less fragmented if the holding environment – in this instance, made up of the network of carers around him or her – is carefully attuned to his or her needs. During the journey of dementia a sense of disintegration might be occurring as a result of the illness. In this stage of unravelling, a good enough holding environment might allow for moments of re-integration, or at least going-on-being – continuity that would provide respite from feelings of existential precariousness. This of course is an aim, since the reality of perfectly adaptable one-to-one care is, as we have seen, short on the ground. Arguably, as perhaps the carers and staff at Winston Grove were advocating, a good holding environment can only be offered when time and resources are available.

In dementia care, we might wonder if an individual's experience of dementia interacts with the level of their pre-existing ego strength. In the communal context of a care home, is it possible that those more able to bear frustrations have had a more fulfilling earlier experience, as we might have seen in Maude? For those with less strong egos pre-dementia, we might imagine the need for closer one-to-one relationships with care staff, the offering of more time. However, for care staff to relate like this, tenderly, intimately, it would be important for them to have the opportunity to think about the sometimes confusing attachment patterns of their clients and possibly their own patterns of relating. These are questions of course for all practitioners working in the field and are beyond the scope of this book.

THE MATRIXIAL

Though the maternal was clearly an important figure in the care home environment, other objects from people's past lives were also important. Daphne herself imagined that her sister, Diane, was in the building; she saw her former partner Benjamin asleep in a chair (when he was no longer visiting); another resident waited patiently at the door for her brother who wasn't coming; Sue remembered her father as well as mother; Maude talked about her husband; Gemma thought about her grandparents, as did Nancy and Prashid too. There was Dorothy's Wendy, and Evie's Johnny, objects for whom no history was known. In other words, there were other figures imagined and reimagined who populated the corridors of both care home sites. From this perspective, Ettinger's (2003) matrixial web provides a rich and helpful theoretical frame to understand what might have been happening both internally and externally at both sites and at different times. The notion of the matrixial also demonstrates why the care home site is such a complex social world to navigate, both as a worker and as someone with dementia, whose temporal horizons keep on shifting.

Borrowing from Ettinger is vital for two reasons: a) because her theoretical model focuses on the pre-verbal experience in utero – this is a point in development which is much earlier on than the focus of those following Klein or Winnicott; b) Ettinger both acknowledges the figure of the maternal as a founding source of the human capacity to share and to co-affect while simultaneously recognising the impact of significant internalised others, also summoned up, in moments of inter-subjective encounter. For her, there are multiple transferences going on between people at any one time, all of which are embedded in an originary experience of co-affecting (which first took place between mother and foetus).

Her work has particular resonance with the dementia care field because it was not just the maternal figure that was in view in both care homes but many others. Though I might argue that mother had the greatest absent-presence, other figures and traces of figures existed in the psychic fields that existed between people. Brothers, sisters, fathers, spouses, and grandparents emerged in speech and were seen in others. All of these important influences interrelated, creating something of a family, or organisational, resonance field (Ettinger, 2006), a psychic landscape made up of deeply embedded memories from divergent family albums.

For Ettinger (2006), whenever 'I' meets with a 'non-I' there is an encounter, which comes to form a particular psychic resonance field. Each field is located with and alongside other fields of resonance. An intricate web of meetings of one within the other, with each meeting belonging to several clusters of fields. The matrixial web is conceptualised as a body-psyche-time-space of the intimate, which is made up of the traces of personal histories that are inhabited by several others. It is from the onset transgressive in so far as human experiences, inner worlds and body worlds, come into contact, overlap. Despite their different theoretical approaches and scholarly preoccupations, there are perhaps echoes in the way that Armstrong's (2005) organisation-in-the-mind ignites the organisation-in-the-mind of others, also considered something of a psychic resonance field. Yet, though the organisation-in-the-mind has been discussed through the lens of the staff, it is the matrixial that seems a more helpful concept in terms of the residents' experiences. The notion of the matrixial is deeply connected to our personal histories, something which is often re-awoken vividly in the journey of dementia and towards death.

I take this to mean that, although each subject is distinct from another, bounded, what takes place in specific encounters between two people, or more, is the evocation of some aspect of the self with all its constitutive objects, memory traces, pre- and unconscious resonances. In dementia care, this sense of many others relating through different spaces and temporal zones seemed tangible. Witnessing this process of losing and finding, transferring and displacing, made transparent the way in which our internal territories can interact with the outside and make new realities. Similarly it made transparent how each individual's internal landscape is mapped out by encounters with significant others who affect and shape our lives, and how our ancestral objects interact with the traces of objects which belong to the well-trodden terrain of others even in an organisational context where interpersonal space is punctuated by role, task, status and projective and defensive processes. (Let us for a moment remember Prashid from Whittinghall reflecting on his grandparents back home.)

What I wish to alert the reader to is that absent (in a physical sense) masculine and feminine identities, family and friends, were enlivened in both care home sites. This is important because I am not suggesting that the care field is only the domain of women or the feminine. On the contrary, the dementia care context is one where myriad fantasised identities exist, are talked about, often (particularly for people with dementia) in an unguarded, non-defensive way – and this allows those in the field to see just how helpful it is to employ both male and female care workers, from a range of ages and indeed backgrounds.

Nonetheless, we must not lose sight of the maternal. I wish to conclude this chapter with Ettinger (2006) in mind because for her the feminine in utero experience (mother's womb) leaves an originary psychic trace of interdependency, impossible to obliterate. It is possible that in our ending days we might at a deeply unconscious level yearn for a return to a space in which an-other encounters us; that in finitude one final holding experience (Winnicott, 1960; 1962) akin to the womb allows us to un-become; that there is some felt presence of a m-other-like-encompassing in the moment of our very absence. Valerie Sinason (1992) so beautifully writes of her client with dementia:

> Edward Johnson had died in his own flat... He was holding his father's
> academic book in one hand and his mother's scarf in the other... once it
> got to the point of the last unravelling, when he knew mindlessness and

death lay ahead, he felt better equipped to go with nature (the tree) and his mother (the scarf) and his father (the book).

(p. 110)

To be clear, I am not likening un-becoming to a process similar to Winnicott's notion of disintegration, although dying fills some people with intolerable levels of fear and panic. Rather, I also envisage a possibility of un-becoming, in a womblike direction, perhaps to my mind, on a par with letting go, or alternatively akin to Barbara Low's Nirvana Principle, which Freud approved of and considered tantamount to the removal of tensions between the life and death drive (Freud, 1949).

DEATH

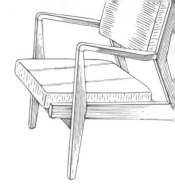

Although death is a very final interruption, there are of course many forms of dying in institutional care that precede the death of the body. We might see this particularly perhaps in terms of 'being dead to' the full experience of others and indeed self; and of 'being deadened' by organisational protocol and procedure. In short, a deadening towards relating – personally or institutionally. Additionally, there seemed to be a real need to find time to do the work of mourning in both organisations. Some staff expressed regret about changes to care practice and to the care environment, and the associated occupational losses; and residents indirectly communicated untold losses of loved ones, home, and cognition.

The organisational culture of both homes had an impact on how people connected and, hence, on how emotionally alive the homes felt. Quite possibly, the number of different types of mother/s that were brought to life, particularly at Winston Grove, spoke of this emotional aliveness. Winston Grove seemed to be the more playful environment and ways into intimacy often consciously involved singing, games, laughing, activity. Winston Grove represented a lively home, although at times this felt like a manic defence against the dying. The number of interruptions I witnessed at Winston Grove seemed to be reflective of this manic functioning. It seemed as if there wasn't – organisationally speaking – a respect for the privacy of bounded beings, who could withdraw into themselves if they needed to do so. It reminded me of the anxious mother constantly checking to see if the newborn was still breathing in his sleep.

At Whittinghall, waiters also entered rooms offering 'biccy biccies' or cups of tea, but interruptions were much fewer. At Whittinghall the environment was palpably deadening at times. Often there was a sense of the heavy futility of human life, watching the world around spin, helpless like Dorothy in the corridor.

Whittinghall tended to represent dying, a waiting space, while for Winston Grove it was active aging. Although this split is too reductive, many factors fed into this general assessment. Winston Grove was an open-planned dementia care site. Residents walked around a lot, and were free to do so. Whittinghall was compartmentalised, in a physical and structural sense, with different units offering different types of care. Though the units were not key-padded, only one male resident, relatively young, crossed the boundary between 'dementia unit' and 'elderly frail'.

At Whittinghall intimate moments of connection were few and far between. When tender encounters did happen they often hinged on the sharing of food, as we see here. Encounters such as this one were also very short-lived.

> Nancy walks past pushing another resident into the hairdresser's office. She walks back to the nurses' station and pulls out a cupcake from somewhere. She walks over to Dorothy and offers her the cake, taking the paper from around it. 'What do I want that for, that for, that for? I don't want that, that, that.' Food: an oral sensation of existing? Dorothy flicks a lot of chocolate topping at Nancy, but then takes the cake, takes a bite of it. Nancy walks back to the nurses' station and sips a drink from a bottle, re-energising? All the while Dorothy has her eyes on her.
>
> The nurse is jotting things down in a file, and the young female carer has her left hand touching the nurse's neck. This is an unexpected moment of intimacy. Between staff.
>
> 'Wendy, Wendy, Wendy,' shouts Dorothy, holding the cake in the air for Nancy.
>
> Nancy walks over, takes a bite and hands it back to Dorothy. Dorothy smiles, taking another bite. Once she has eaten that one she calls out again, 'Wendy, Wendy, Wendy,' holding up the cake again. Eating, drinking, usually connects them.
>
> Nancy pretends to take a bite then hands the cake back. 'No, no, no more,' says Dorothy. Nancy takes the cake and throws it in the bin behind the station. Enough play for today.
>
> (Whittinghall)

Connection, intimacy, and disconnection relate either to the capacity to be alive to other people or to the need to close off to them (to be dead to…). One formulation was that the more regulated a care site, the less scope there was for taking risks in the relating and getting it wrong. Care became more professionalised, which led to a more distanced, deadening sense of relating.

The sense of disconnection present in Whittinghall could be seen and felt in a range of factors: uniforms created clear demarcations between residents and staff, not so at Winston Grove; Dorothy was not free to move and often care staff would put the brakes on her wheelchair, whereas Daphne walked everywhere; and the nurses' station at Whittinghall was a designated space for staff to do their work in, whereas at Winston Grove staff members sat side by side with residents, filling in care plans. Huntside was also designated 'elderly frail', which seemed to enhance its overall sense of paralysis. Given that Winston Grove was a home specifically for people with dementia, it is unsurprising that there were more people with advanced cases of dementia there. Interestingly, Whittinghall felt more deadening even though some people in Dorothy's unit were mentally alert. This lifelessness was captured in the image of Dorothy stuck in the corridor, the residents in bed behind closed doors.

That is not to say Whittinghall was wholly without life. There was, for instance, a resident who was excited at the thought of a protest at the end of a corridor; another who made demands for more wine at lunch. These two residents suggested that life, and agency, were represented in the home, though possibly not as well tolerated as at Winston Grove. Nevertheless, its deadened atmosphere was palpable. The organisational response to failing health was to erect fairly rigid procedures, to compartmentalise roles. At one point a tablet care-planning device was introduced, seemingly another example of tidying the place up, managing efficiently but rather inhumanely. A sense of stasis and unimaginative interaction between residents and staff also often ensued. Here Dorothy tries to get attention, again to no avail. As a result, she withdraws into herself, a symbol of social death.

'Can you hear me, can you hear me?' Dorothy says. She drops her head down and rests her chin on her right hand. Heavy again. She stays in that position, looking down at her stomach, her breath up and down. She half-closes her eyes.

The phone is going. No one is answering it.

Nancy walks into the corridor. She looks tired. She talks about time passing, summer ending, autumn beginning soon. The new system. All members of staff are carrying devices, tablets. Each person can note down episodes of residents' care as they go, on the job, tapping on icons to record information about different types of care – food, hair, teeth. At the moment

*staff seem unsettled by the development, but soon they might come to like
their phone devices.*

(Whittinghall)

The other feature of Whittinghall was the apparent cut-offness of the
residents. It was very rare to see residents walking around the home,
particularly upstairs in Dorothy's unit. The same was true of lunchtimes
in which the large dining room was barely used. Tables were left empty
with only a few residents ever making use of the social space.

This is Peter, one resident who spent each and every day in his room,
as many others did:

PETER

*Peter was a man who kept himself to himself. His room was very
comfortable, with photos of his daughter on a mantelpiece, an image of
him, younger, by a line of boats. The television was on in Peter's room,
very loud, with something like* Antiques in the Attic *on. Peter was
lying in bed, a cotton sheet pulled up to his chest. He had a white shirt
on underneath. He was chatty and welcoming. He laughed a lot. Despite
the seeming liveliness of the laughter, Peter seemed stuck in his room,
in his bed.*

*Peter is daydreaming. 'I could do it on my own. I will do it. I'll just buzz
off somewhere… Devon, Cornwall, anywhere. Since the time I've lived
here, not seeing anybody. But uh. [The telephone is buzzing in the corridor
but no one is picking up.] Unless I meet a young lady and she has plenty
of money… I'd say that'd be nice. I'll have your money and we can buzz off.'
Peter is laughing but there is a tragedy in this life, as he knows this is not
possible. 'We all want to do it.' Peter is silent. 'I don't think that would ever
happen though…' (Silence again). 'I don't think that'll ever happen… go
face there. That's it.' (Silence). 'Don't know. Apart from that, you know…
that's it, isn't it really? Well when you live here like I do you think well,
what shall I do today? Well… that's no good to me… that's it. Well. Like
to go to Devon or somewhere, travel around a bit. But uh… I wouldn't sort
of sit here and think of… I'd just do something or whatever…That's it…
but um. You know, that's it. You know. I don't want to meet some old girl
just for her money. She can keep her ruddy money. Think hello hello, she's
after my loot. Which has all gone… But uh there we are. Well uh it's all
right sitting here like this innit, sitting here, watching your toes go up and*

down.' He looks at his feet underneath the cover and moves his toes up and down. 'Yeah, watch your toes thing.'

(Whittinghall)

The pain of Peter's isolation was intense at times. He seemed preoccupied by money, mentioning it over twenty times, and by finding a companion (whom he feared would take his money). Money would allow him to find the companion, and also help him to escape. Yet, on some level, Peter recognised these were pipedreams, which made his predicament all the more depressing. 'That's it,' he uttered several times as if it were 'game over'. I noticed myself feeling marginally uncomfortable, sensing a low-level erotic transference. But watching Peter, under cover, television booming, heightened the pain of loneliness and the inevitable slowing-down of life, of desire. At Whittinghall, there seemed to be an absence of the possibility for play and, though death was discussed with staff, the home did not offer the residents the possibility of mourning their losses. The environment tended to be sterile, and this had seeped into the resident experience. Dorothy was for ever wiping crumbs from her top as if nothing could be out of place.

Peter's stuckness in the room was hard to be around, despite his performance of jollity. Finally, when he talks about lying in his bed watching his toes go up and down, the full weight of this deadening paralysis could be felt. Peter seemed to represent something about the risks involved in being alive to an-other. He imagines being together with a woman, but that togetherness is tinged with a fear that connection leads to loss (in his case 'loot'). This seemed to mirror the sense of Whittinghall, where carers remained at a distance, perhaps partially conscious that deep attachments were too emotionally costly in the face of death. Or perhaps, being a privately run home, the staff imagined they had to be more business-like, professional; that the concept of care was intertwined more closely with notions of service provision, of having customers.

The unbearable nature of this heavy isolation each week was exemplified in the haunting voices of Dorothy or Evie calling out for 'Wendy' or 'Johnny' repetitively. What made it harder was noticing these cries going unheard, ignored. This meant that Dorothy and Evie were almost always alone with the experience of a lost object, which could not be brought to life creatively either through memory or simple conversation with a member of staff. One particular observation was striking. Not only was Evie left to look after herself, but she was given a cup that read 'Funeral Directors'. The link between the absence of caring relationships and an acute sense of death in the residents' social world was poignant.

Evie is calling out, 'Johnny, Johnny.' Every now and then she pushes herself forward slightly and grabs a piece of toast with marmalade on it, taking a bite. 'Ooh, ooh, ooh,' she calls out after finishing her bite. She is slumped down low in her chair; it is as if the armchair is swallowing her up. Her loose skin falls around her neck, which seems almost weighted down by it. 'Johnny, Johnny,' she says. Her cup of tea branded 'Funeral Directors'. Sometimes you might think there are subliminal messages everywhere.

'Sit upright, sit upright,' Evie tells herself. Evie is parenting herself, it's painful to witness.

(Whittinghall)

Interestingly Nancy and Sonia, the senior nurse, explained how residents sometimes decided they were ready to die in Whittinghall. Perhaps this made sense of Peter's self-exclusion there; there was doubtless some truth in both Sonia's and Nancy's assertions that many residents had chosen to stay in their bedrooms. This had to be acknowledged, but I also knew that Dorothy shut herself in whenever she felt rejected.

Sonia was very thoughtful about what she had experienced with dying residents. Her willingness to try to engage with the emotional component of her work, trying to understand what this did to her, surprised me. This seemed to be in contrast with the professionalised distance of many Whittinghall staff. It dawned on me that perhaps part of the distance I experienced, in Sonia's unit (Huntside), at least, had to do with the fact that the team at times handled palliative cases. In fact, they were conscious of palliative work in a way that Winston Grove didn't seem to be. The preparation for death that Sonia notes might well have involved a necessary cutting off.

Sonia is methodical in her approach. '... some people they think oh that resident is in their room... and don't want to do anything. It's not like that. Some residents are very very old and just want to rest. We have Evie and she was here in the morning and we try to make her walk and we take her, because it is better for her, out of her room. But what she really likes, if you'd let her, she would stay in her bed all day. But her family don't want her to do that. So sometimes she will sit in a chair for a long while and then she'll ask to go to bed and if it's what she really wants and she is more comfortable there then… She feels tired. We can't just take her to do things if she doesn't want to…' Sonia may be responding to criticisms that Huntside has received. 'You can't just come here and expect to see everybody doing something. Some of them just don't want to do anything else. And it's hard as well to see, when we… we know a resident for a while and we have someone that used to be active and do things and were interested. And suddenly they just give up. It happened before. It's hard for us to see that… And with dementia you just won't ever get better you tend to get worse, and it's really difficult for them to accept that. Sometimes you have to deal with the resident and with the family as well.' The care staff's lot is not easy, not easy at all. 'Very difficult when we have a resident who gives up and they say "I think it's my time"; "I'm not doing anything else, I just want to go, I am tired of living." This is hard for us to hear as well because when we know them and we saw how they were before… so I can understand for the family it is even worse. But we have to respect that and we can't force them.' 'To keep on living?' I ask. Sonia tells a story of a man she remembers. 'This happened before. We had a resident and he said that he wanted to live just to celebrate his eighty-fifth birthday. He came here, he was fine. He had a big party. And after a couple of months, maybe two months, he began to deteriorate… He stopped eating, and um he seemed more depressed and he said that he wanted to go. And yeah he did. And it happened. He just said that he didn't want to live anymore, he'd had enough… When we are expecting a death we kind of prepare ourselves… Sometimes we think oh it's just work but it's not a work where we deal with machines, we deal with emotions. And when we deal with the emotions of someone else we need to deal with the emotions of ourselves and it's not easy. And sometimes we need a break, a holiday, just to focus on something else to recover and come back but if we like what we do we manage to do it.'

(Whittinghall)

Speaking to Sonia suggested that Whittinghall's pervasive sense of deadness did not simply stem from a proceduralised and inflexible culture, one in which capacities for connection and thinking were minimised. Nancy had also explained that she tried not to get too attached to residents, for fear of them dying. It hurt. Things that hurt are often avoided. Perhaps the cost of engaging with residents who were increasingly withdrawing from life was too great. I began to wonder how the young staff team were supported organisationally to process the deaths they encountered. Apart from informal chats, hugs, and holidays, which Sonia spoke of, there didn't seem to be anything in place to process loss.

Winston Grove was, at least on the surface, quite different. During my observations there, I was frequently struck by my counter-transference – a feeling of being on edge in the face of loud music, whooping sounds to the hoopla. The lively atmosphere also jarred with the slouched bodies of residents trying to sleep through the noise and laughter. I came to think this was an organisational denial of, a manic flight away from, the nameless and inevitable pull of death, which was in the home yet spoken nowhere.

Although taking a different form from Whittinghall, anxiety around both physical and social death was also defended against at Winston Grove. In the final visit, Diane talked about the funeral of Daphne's long-term partner, Benjamin, who had died the week before, as if this were just another of Daphne's trips out. Though Daphne's anxiety was at a very heightened level that day, the home keeps going – active, alive – and the response to her psychic pain was to take her out to the local coffee shop. The quiet solitude Daphne might have needed was well out of reach.

Today she is sitting at a dining table. Diane is explaining to Daphne that she is giving her her medication. 'I don't know what to do,' says Daphne. 'Open your mouth, Daphne, and I will pop this in your mouth,' she says, pointing to a tablet. Daphne opens her mouth and the carer gently places the spoon and tablets inside. She screws her face up. Diane hands Daphne a glass of water and asks her to drink it all down. She looks up at the carer, and smiles at her.

This is care; the everyday realities of making sure people keep on going; the everyday realities of watching people become more dependent. Newborns, fledgling birds, old, old people opening their mouths and waiting for some kind of care. Life's circle closing, closing in.

Elaine's dog, Screech, walks in to the dining area and stands at the doors that face out onto the garden. 'Oh, hello there,' says Daphne. 'You want to go out Screech?' says Diane to the dog. Daphne pushes herself up from her chair and walks towards the door and stands close behind the carer. 'Bye bye,' she says to the dog, endings in her mind. 'Bye bye.'

Daphne is wearing a grey floral blouse, a grey cardigan, black skirt, black socks, black shoes. She has on her purple tinted glasses. She stands by the door for some time and watches the carer go into the kitchen. Daphne looks at me, sadly. 'I don't even know who I am,' she says, and it's hard to think about what Daphne says without thinking of Benjamin and the meaning that his existence had given her. 'I don't know what to do.' The dog reappears at the door, and Diane notices. She stops by the door and opens it up. 'Back already?' she says.

Daphne makes a noise as if she is in pain. It is a quivering sound. 'I don't know what to do, where I am. I want my parents,' she says, looking around the room. Lost children, in lost continents.

Daphne walks into the room where Gemma and another carer, Celia, are getting residents ready to go out.

'Their worlds don't understand my world; my world doesn't understand theirs,' says Daphne. 'They are too busy. They can't pay attention to you.' She begins to make this quivering, anxious noise again, holding her hands together tightly around her. You imagine Daphne is falling apart inside. She begins to stare at an empty chair, loss, while Celia is getting one woman ready. This woman doesn't have a coat in her bedroom and so Celia sacrifices hers for now. 'Is that okay?' The woman puts on the carer's coat and seems delighted. 'Oh well very well then,' she says. 'How wonderful this is.'

'I think all I can do is sit down,' says Daphne. She goes to a chair, stands over it but doesn't sit down. She walks back towards the carer, Diane, who is now speaking with Suki who seems to have changed her mind about going out. Daphne is watching. 'Help me, help me,' she says in a quiet voice.

'What will I do then?' she asks. 'Well you are going out on Thursday,' says Diane to Daphne, but going out we know is for Benjamin's funeral. This is not for leisure. 'I want to come with you,' says Daphne to Diane.

'Well I am staying here with you, Daphne, and we can make some tea together and eat some custard creams.'

'Oh good,' says Daphne. 'I don't really know what to do. Can we help each other?' Daphne is clutching at people and you wonder if this is because she knows, deep down, that she has just lost Benjamin.

(Winston Grove)

It is as if Daphne is dying inside here. It was impossible for the carers to attend to Daphne in the way she needed. The carers were busy, carrying out the physical tasks involved in a trip out on a cold day. The emotional and psychic turmoil that Daphne was experiencing had little place, in that moment. She needed someone present to her 'world', one that was increasingly incomplete. Daphne had an ability to communicate exactly what was going on for her, and when she looks at the empty chair it is as if she knows that there has been a death, one that makes her feel as if she too is unravelling, empty.

This observation was a very difficult one because I also knew that I would be leaving Winston Grove, as my visits had come to an end. Daphne had already lost a major attachment in Benjamin, not only an attachment to love and connection, but also to the outside world and her past. The loss was tremendous and leaving her worried me, imagining that each empty space and chair at Winston Grove would represent yet another death for Daphne.

Gemma, the activities co-ordinator, arguably represented a denial of death for the organisation. After all, being so close to grief, the impact of a death could be very disturbing. The activities Gemma led were boisterous and had an air of celebration. What follows is Daphne's struggle to join in, in need of something calmer, some peace.

A pile of books has been pulled out of the bookshelf, discarded on the floor. Daphne is in the toilet, the door is wide open. This was the all-hanging-outness of Winston Grove. A member of staff appears, closing the door gently, seeing that Daphne's privacy is at stake.

Daphne emerges from the toilet. She is fiddling with her fingers, worried. 'It is a concern that the children are here without their parents.' Thinking about how they will be looked after is making her nervous. She is concerned about her mother, too. 'Although,' she says, 'I suppose I could stop myself just there and look at her.' She stares outside at the fountain for some time then turns to me. 'Perhaps if you think it would be okay, I could come and help you do what you do.' She hasn't seen that she is helping me now.

Bitterly cold outside, despite the sun's rays, Daphne is dressed in a warm cardigan and a blue floral blouse which ties – a loose ribbon – around her neck. She begins walking. There is no one in reception today. Daphne stops, looks around, and keeps going past the unit where she has her breakfast, towards loud music dating back to the 'forties. She stands at the edge of the double doors to another lounge, watching, cautious.

A man is throwing hoops at the target in front of him. There are about fifteen residents there, most in chairs. Some are clapping in time with the music and others mouthing the words, 'Goodbye Piccadilly, farewell Leicester Square'.

Daphne is observing. 'I don't want to look silly today,' she says, explaining that she tries her best not to be a stupid old woman. It hurts to hear this. She wants something 'quiet' today, as if she is conscious that her social world is shrinking further out of reach; as if conscious that she is losing the Daphne able to filter the appropriate from the inappropriate. The fear of doing something shameful leads to her self-exclusion. She goes back to her regular lounge. She sits, squeezing her hands together, as if holding on to some semblance of Daphne, to self.

(Winston Grove)

Speaking with Gemma, it became clear that she felt the experience of being dependent in a care home could lead to a meaningless existence. She seemed preoccupied with 'doing' as a way of remedying this futility. She wanted residents to retain their capacity for activity. Doing was a marker of life.

Smiling, she said, 'I kind of deal with the social life of residents with dementia... trying to keep them motivated. Have a purpose in life... keep them busy really... trying to keep them going [large sigh], I suppose. 'Cos if it was me and I'd been put in a home... well not everybody wants to go in a care home, it might be better for some of them because they were... social isolation.'

(Two work men walk in and start moving a chair in the background then walk out.)

'Well for me if I'd been put in a care home... and they're just... I don't know... you have your lunch... you get up... you have your lunch at this time... It's something to keep you... You'd be like "why am I living? What's my point?" So it's something to keep you going... Do what you used to do. Going out for walks, as we have done today. Um... and not just being sat in a chair to fall asleep in front of the TV all day and cabbage out. Life doesn't end just because you've come in a care home, I don't think.'

(Winston Grove)

Gemma's attachment to residents' past abilities is an interesting phenomenon – perhaps symbolic of the organisation's struggle with allowing mourning. This is one possible set of meanings. Another might be that by holding tightly on to former identities, the changing self can neither be fully borne nor accommodated by the organisation, although observations generally suggested that care staff tried to adapt to the residents' changes. Nonetheless the avoidance of mourning, dependency, loss, and death was striking; so much so that death – the word – was not mentioned by any single interviewee at Winston Grove.

It was striking that Sonia and Nancy had broached the subject of dying as sensitively as they had done. It left me with questions: what does death stir up in workers? How difficult is it to accept the failure involved in letting someone go? What about compassion fatigue and how does an organisation support being over doing? Addressing death explicitly as a national policy issue is of course a vital issue for end-of-life practitioners and for care homes across the country.

Around the theme of death I could see that both care homes were imperfect and both had some good qualities. There was in Winston Grove the possibility for spontaneity and aliveness, where identities could show themselves easily and make stands, yet the home didn't always offer the privacy and solitude needed by those who were increasingly dependent or dying (socially or physically). Whittinghall's professionalised manner created a compliant culture in which complaints were swallowed down with biccies, as if the biscuits could medicate away ill-feeling. Possibly, though, the quiet distancing in Whittinghall afforded some residents a calm in which the long rest could finally take place.

The distanced mode of relating found in Whittinghall made room for some capacity to look death in the eye, which the manic activity in Winston Grove did not permit. Winston Grove took risks in human relating, which allowed people to be heard a little louder and to be seen with greater complexity.

Winston Grove generally felt like an alive home, although this aliveness was tinged with mania, quite possibly a systemic defence against the fear of death. Being forced into life (through singing, bingo, dancing, painting, joking) and into living was not always appropriate, and seemed to prevent staff at Winston Grove from thinking about the unbearableness of loss. It was possible that denying death served a purpose: in maintaining a fantasy that the residents could be kept alive through the provision of good care, this might have meant that carers put considered effort into relating intimately with those in their care, ensuring they knew all the small details that made things better for individuals. The other side of this denial, though, was that staff at Winston Grove did not seem able to reflect upon experiences of separation, endings, and loss as some did at Whittinghall.

Represented in Gemma, the activities co-ordinator, there were moments of a manic triumphalism, and denial, over death, as seen in her comment during an exercise session. She moves very fast, but jokingly criticises the residents for going slowly, like 'wet lettuces'. Finally, when Benjamin had died, no one was able to broach his death with Daphne. The whole issue was swept under the carpet; Daphne was taken on a trip to a busy local cafe, with other residents, in response to her mounting levels of anxiety.

The environment at Whittinghall, on the contrary, felt deadening. Peter's toes going up and down in his bed, alone in his room, bored, paralysed, watching *Antiques in the Attic*, symbolised an organisational lack of liveliness.

The sterile, still environment at Whittinghall was partly due to the absence each day of residents wandering freely around, the absence of freedom outside the confines of the routine. The neat compartmentalised and compartmentalising culture meant that residents were unable to live spontaneously alongside one another and the staff leading it seemed oblivious to these minute-by-minute social deaths. Nonetheless this socially frozen organisational culture seemed to give people space to withdraw into themselves in order to retreat into death. Alternatively, there were moments when I wondered if organisationally Whittinghall was not capable of generating life, the expectation being that people would die.

I also wondered if the pervasive presence of death – especially given the palliative cases at Huntside – meant that staff distanced themselves from getting close, from becoming too vulnerable to loss. Balfour (2006) describes a difficult staff supervision group within a staff team in a hospital, who were attempting to process the 'tremendous painfulness of the work, that good work often meant helping people to die'. The painfulness that Balfour depicts may have been one of the reasons why staff adopted more professionalised modes of relating. Whittinghall's approach to death was noticeably different to a palliative care model of death, though, which takes on a more existential approach: one in which caring for dying people is seen to provide rich opportunities for connection and the discovery of meanings. In essence, it seemed that death anxieties were inarticulate in different ways within each organisation. In the face of death, there were very different organisational reactions. However, as Klein argued in her (1940/1975) formulation of mourning, building on Freud's *On Murder, Mourning and Melancholia* (1917/2005), we might begin to see that a far-reaching anxiety about the residents (old age and dementia possibly experienced as persecutory) may have underpinned the defensive responses to the dying context.

In 'Mourning and its Relation to Manic-Depressive States', Klein (1940) shows how the work of mourning involves the reactivation of the original depressive position in which the infant, at the point of weaning, feels the loss of the good breast, experienced as damaged by his own greed and aggression (1940, p. 345). This fear of losing loved objects owing to one's own destructive thoughts and impulses repeats throughout the life course, according to Klein, particularly in relation to parents and to siblings. Her contention was that, in the process of normal mourning, anxieties about having destroyed real loved objects are reignited. In normal mourning, the adult would be working from a place of a secure internal world in which 'good' objects were brought into the ego and restored during the depressive phase, where one can accept both one's loving and hating feelings. In other words, the depressive position successfully worked through provides a prototype for normal mourning later on.

At both Whittinghall and Winston Grove, there was possibly a pervasive difficulty with the process of normal mourning. I turn to Klein:

> *The fundamental difference between normal mourning on the one hand, and abnormal mourning and manic-depressive states on the other, is this: the manic-depressive and the person who fails in the work of mourning, though their defences may differ widely from each other, have this in common, that they have been unable in early childhood to establish their internal good objects and to feel secure in their inner world. They have never really overcome the infantile depressive position... It is by reinstating inside himself the 'good' parents as well as the recently lost person, and by rebuilding his world, which was disintegrated and in danger, that he overcomes grief, regains security and achieves true harmony and peace.*
>
> (p. 369)

At Winston Grove and Whittinghall, I am talking about the psychic life of the organisation as a whole (Obholzer & Zagier Roberts, 1994; Armstrong & Huffington, 2004), and am not suggesting that both care homes were populated by staff who had not worked through the depressive position. Chaya and Ursula, for instance, were both able to mourn and to integrate apparently contradictory ideas. This is not about pathologising care workers in any way. However, if we are to take on board Klein's idea that the depressive anxieties, of damaging and the associated guilt, reactivated each time there is a significant loss in someone's life, and we know that this is not an easy position to work through, in the first instance, without a backdrop of ongoing love and support, we might surmise that working closely with people who will die poses workers with the permanent threat of having their internal worlds destabilised.

As noted already, Winston Grove had a particularly lively quality of activity, and sometimes an 'obsessional nature of the impulses to reparation' (p. 353) which were ways of mastering the anxiety that the staff had in relation to being close to dying residents. Equally, Whittinghall could have been regarded as obsessional in its control of the residents' freedoms, as symbolised in the regularity with which Dorothy's wheelchair brakes were put on. Beyond this, there was a marked example of idealisation in the interview from Chaya, and towards the organisation itself from Nancy, Sonia, and Prashid, which defended against reflecting on the toll of the work. Klein notes that,

Idealisation is an essential part of the manic position and is bound up with another important element of that position, denial. Without partial and temporary denial of psychic reality the ego cannot bear the disaster by which it feels itself threatened when the depressive position is at its height. Omnipotence, denial and idealisation, closely bound up with ambivalence, enable the early ego to assert itself to a certain degree against its internal persecutors and against a slavish and perilous dependence upon its loved objects and thus to make further advances in development.

(p. 349)

Although Winston Grove and Whittinghall reacted very differently towards death, it does seem possible that without the opportunity to do some meaningful thinking about loss, it was difficult for individuals to rebuild their inner worlds, or to integrate ambivalences, characteristic of the successful process of mourning. I wish to leave this section on death with the pertinent words of Daphne who said the following:

> So that in itself has brought this to life so although it doesn't seem totally full in the world today there, it clearly is part of it and it does tell part of its part to other people there so they can get used to things for themselves. And start talking about their experience rather than where it is or how old it was and didda dada um bombom...

(Winston Grove).

Daphne seemed to understand that the experiences of being in a care home were multi-layered and that it was important to speak about being in an intermediate place not 'full in the world', one in which moments of joy in living existed side by side with the fear of dying. Not full in the world because the residents were also moving out of the world. Trying to understand and to tolerate this (transitional) space of life and death seemed to be important for residents and staff alike, even though for the most part there was a need, it seemed, to keep such thoughts out of conscious awareness.

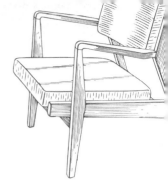

FINAL WORDS

'You cannot rush care; you cannot compromise care.'
Celia, 24 March 2015, Winston Grove

Writing the final words to this exploration of dementia care is almost as difficult as saying goodbye to Daphne, to Dorothy, to Melie, to all the residents whom I have had the privilege to spend time with. As a professional carer, as I once was, the people you care about, and for, sometimes hold on to you as you try to end your shift. In my case, even today, residents hold on through the hauntings of memory. Saying goodbye in dementia care is one of the most challenging parts of the work, when all has gone well and a friendship has formed. A carer can become for a resident, as Nancy had been during those early weeks with Dorothy, an anchor in all the confusion. A carer might know that saying goodbye will disrupt, dislocate, and unsettle those s/he cares for, and yet to carry on doing the work s/he has to pull away. Opening up to the experiences of other people, good and bad, can be engulfing and sometimes debilitating. Time and space to refuel is essential. Yet at home, after a busy day, a carer might continue to think about a Daphne or a Dorothy, and become anxious that some component of the work was left undone, that at some point she was unable to help put back together someone in distress. So she is left distressed herself, guilty. On other days, the joy of sharing a moment, arranging napkins for the lunch table while laughing about the imperfection of the triangular-shaped folds you've done together, provides a sense of meaning and reward.

I am struck by what the existential psychotherapist Yalom (2008) might describe as 'rippling'. Dreamily written, his book uses the ripples in a pond as an analogy for the way each of us creates 'concentric circles of influences that may affect others for years, for generations' (p83). I know that residents and carers with whom I have worked will continue to have some impact on the way I steer my life.

Both care home sites were imperfect places. Winston Grove had the quality of being at times both managed and unmanageable in the sense that the manager cared and got involved, but that some of the very difficult feelings within the organisation couldn't be harnessed and reflected upon. Often those who had a valency for anger and anxiety were not embraced in the same way that more grateful, playful residents and staff were. Like the social policy context, the emotional complexity of the work could be avoided. Yet there was something warm and community-spirited about Winston Grove, which simultaneously made room for risk-taking and spontaneity, both important factors in creating and preserving relatedness.

Whittinghall was quite different. The neat luxurious surrounds meant that people were physically comfortable and staff knew more clearly where their roles began and ended. The procedural management of the home, and related compartmentalisation, meant that contact with residents and staff was more distanced, colder. Yet this distance provided an opportunity to acknowledge more openly the reality that people would die. There was not the manically defended functioning – the parties, the frequent noisy activity, the animal life – found at Winston Grove, but rather lots of quiet space. This quiet space was double-edged. It may have been needed for those receiving end of life care, but for many residents this quiet possibly reinforced the painful isolation of being out of mind and out of home.

The real absence in both sites, though, was the formal or informal space for staff teams to be able to process the work they were doing. It seemed clear that the people who worked in both sites were at times filled up with the emotional labour of the work. Diane felt brutalised by its relentlessness and, interview over, Bridget discussed her continued anxiety about an incident that had happened years before around the breakfast table. Nancy explained that she would have to leave Whittinghall when Dorothy died because they had become close against all odds; and Sophia knew that touching death in her work made her reach out to life – and to holidays.

Because neither organisation provided a space for a more reflective kind of practice, staff inevitably held much in. Social care policy is behind in its thinking about the support of and identities of staff teams. National palliative care policy is more developed in its understanding of the unmet needs of its workers. For instance, in March 2015, Hospice UK launched its framework, *Resilience*, for supporting staff teams in hospices, particularly to mitigate stress. Here supervision, training, and compassion fatigue are considered in some detail. There is a focus on fostering a culture in which honest conversations within organisations can take place. Even in the *End of Life Care* Strategy, published in 2008, just before *Living Well: A National Dementia Strategy*, there is some acknowledgement that care staff might be distressed by the work (p. 53) and that reflective practice is beneficial (pp. 66, 140). It also explicitly states that the work involves 'physical, social, psychological and spiritual' (pp. 7, 28, 33, 82, 95, 120, 160) components.

In borrowing from psychoanalytical thinkers, not only can we come to better understand the dementia care field, but we find that there are actual practices that might help us to better support it, too. Staff, like residents, need to be held. Holding, in a Winnicottian sense, involves the simple yet challenging process of being heard, of making room for the bearing witness of experience by an-other who is able to sit with the full range of emotional content. This is not skills training, which involves a seeming expert offering up theory or fact to those not in the know. The work of psychoanalytically informed reflection is about the connections and meanings that can be formed in and through a process of jointness-in-differentiation (Ettinger, 2006).

This all sounds too abstract, I would argue, which is why in the end I might turn to Bion, who made it clear that we learn about ourselves, or, in this case, about ourselves in our work, through a steady process of reflecting upon emotional experience alongside others. This is an intimate act. Learning is not about theorising here, but about carefully unwrapping ourselves, exploring the act of avoiding Dorothy as she cried out; of forcing Melie to brush her teeth; of bringing Daphne to bingo when she is tearful; of turning a corner when Suki needs the toilet... exploring the feeling behind these acts honestly and in such a way as to be able to recognise our imperfect humanness, our failings. This then allows room for thought, the rational and logical. This is not about getting it right, but rather about being able to find a third space within the work that allows teams to recognise the pulls and pushes of the work, without relying on rigidly defensive and protective practice, and without withdrawing. It allows something generative to take place where connections form in the mind and then in the work and back again. This is about finding a space (and a protected space which ripples through the culture) within the institution, where 'meanings can be discovered... In the third space, the meanings of the situation can be explored. What are the areas of generativity? The short answer is thinking and thought... the capacity to think is the major asset of the people in any enterprise.' (Lawrence, 1994, p. 94, cited in Foster, 2010)

To do this successfully in care institutions, policy must notice the emotional cost of the work, it must recognise the 'who' of its workers. Time must be allocated to listening and to feeling and to thinking. Further research into processes of supervision – which give thought to the emotional toll of care work and the way this intersects with categories of class, race, gender – and the impact on daily practice, and intimate relating, is imperative. We are also talking about monetary investment to provide the resources and time within a shift to do so; about the leadership taking an active role in supporting the psychological going-on-being of the team; and an investment in the relational which at least matches the technical and procedural investment.

Class and race

As I have alluded to earlier, race and class were also issues which tended to be pushed out of the organisations' conscious awareness.

When talking with Bridget, the cleaner, and Diane, the carer, I noticed how (socially constructed) categories of class and race seemed to have got inside both women to shape who they were, their subjectivities. This subjective quality, in turn, was one that, I felt sure, had an impact on our conversations. During observations I also noticed the diverse backgrounds of both carers and residents, how at times there were very obvious differences between the older people and their carers. In Whittinghall residents were generally very affluent yet workers were not well paid; residents were elderly and staff members were in their twenties; in Winston Grove the people with dementia tended to be white-skinned and many workers were black-skinned. As such, confused power dynamics and competition were often observed. These power dynamics interacted with the punctuation of interpersonal space, through the boundaries of role and task. For Bridget, she inflated her authority within the organisation, quite possibly in protest against the class category she felt she had been assigned to in life, and relatedly against the role she had been employed to do within the organisation. Diane pushed against the task of time-driven personal care, possibly in resistance to the management which she experienced as a brutalising, abusive one. These differences were palpable in both sites, differences saturated with social power.

I remember one resident at Whittinghall, a Dr Jesmond, who very much related to the staff team as 'service providers', clear that he was a paying guest, entitled to make demands for wine. In the minds of the staff team, though, he was not a consumer but a vulnerable older man. There was also Suki, who repeated that her son was a doctor, educated and professional, in contrast to her reluctant carer, who nonetheless had the power to get Suki to the toilet on time or not; and there was Diane's harrowing recollection of enduring racist abuse at work while understanding that she was in charge of her abuser's care and could therefore be accused of abuse herself. These kinds of issues were often kept out of mind in the daily work of the care home site, and so I feel it is vital to say a little about how 'deep and injurious the impact' (Ryan, 2014, p.133) of being defined by categories such as race and class can be and how resentment might leak into the work, disconnection ensuing, if it is not thought about.

Third spaces in practice and policy

I have been much inspired by Frank Lowe's (2014) book, *Thinking Space*, which followed his initiative at the Tavistock Clinic to create a forum offering a 'container for thought' (2014, p. x), one in which race and other differences were taken seriously enough to encourage an organisational curiosity about difference, rather than shutting it down and splitting it off.

Joanna Ryan (2014) writes, in her exploratory study on class in the consulting room, about the way that 'class and class difference can enter into and contribute to the structuring of the transference–counter-transference matrix...' (p. 127). She discusses the difficulty that therapists reported in speaking of class openly in their relationships with clients despite the class-related transferences and counter transferences experienced; she also understood this repression as being a manifestation of the anxieties around what Layton (2004, cited in Ryan, 2014) describes as the 'internalisation of class relations' (p. 129).

To think of Armstrong (2005), Bridget's organisation-in-the-mind was indeed populated with categories of hierarchy that were seemingly crafted by local government, and which led to splits and the punctuation of interpersonal space around both role and task.

Bridget represented a sort of inverse snobbery where I became unknowing and useless ('education gets you nowhere') while she had all the answers. Bridget made it clear that her position within the organisational, and social, structure did not preclude her from thinking, and this was certainly the case. She had a lot of wisdom. It was as if there was a reversal of the inequalities that she may have experienced outside of the care home or even within it, even within our conversation, in which I certainly began to feel less knowing than she was. A similar feeling was evoked in me with Celia, which I have touched upon earlier. I only wish to say that with both women there were moments where I felt, as a middle-class (defined societally rather than personally) person with a degree, that I was the incompetent one. It was hard to tease apart how much these dynamics related to an anxiety about our different social statuses or whether it was simply the case that, organisationally, in this instance, Bridget and Celia did in reality have the most important knowledge (the histories of residents).

However, I could not help but wonder if perhaps the psychic pain of powerlessness and inequality that these women endured in relation to more affluent residents (the home was in a middle class ward of the London borough) had had an impact on the way that they took up power in our conversations. I wonder now in retrospect how these wide discursive categories, which shape subjectivities and construct subjects, influence the way that people relate to one another in the care home site.

What race has in common with class is that it is another 'term … used to sort varieties of humankinds. Implicit in this possibility is the apparent truism that *there are indeed different kinds of humans to be sorted*' (Dalal, 2002, p. 9). There is little room here to take up a detailed exploration of race and class in dementia care, although I think it important to acknowledge Rustin's view (1991, cited in Dalal, 2002, p. 10) that '"race" is an empty category filled with different sorts of projection and that notions of race can serve a worrying function: the function is the naturalisation of power relations by retaining the divisions of humankind' (p. 13). These socially constructed differences, and divisions, presented by some as the natural order within humankind, are implicitly considered effects of wider power relations, and the discourses they entertain.

Simultaneously, I wish to suggest – in line with Frank Lowe's work – that for someone like Diane who seemed to feel herself to be positioned as a racialised other, a denial of the way that race (Lewis, 2009) had made its mark on her life, and in her work, seemed to make her feel isolated and further brutalised.

As I listened to Diane, and she pointed out that she wasn't the 'right person to talk to', because, ostensibly, her account was not a flattering one, I wondered whether she felt I might also reject her words, in the same way that her stories of racism had been rejected by the senior team. Was I no good, allied with the white manager of the home, who put a stop to hearing Diane's experience? Or was I allied with the white residents, who attacked her care? Or was she no good, as a black woman, whose material didn't fit an idealising script? I had no answers to these questions. What became clear, though, as Diane's powerful interview was disrupted, interrupted by a senior carer, was how easily thinking about race and its effects on the experience of working in the care home was dismissed. Organisationally race was ignored as a factor affecting the caring experience at Winston Grove (and enacted in the counter-transference), and it was not mentioned at all at Whittinghall. Furthermore, the historical backdrop, so important in forming Diane's experience and quite possibly that of the resident whom she described as surviving the Holocaust, were disregarded, which suggested that at times residents and workers were seen only through the lens of the immediate care task, or the routine, in hand.

Without developing thinking spaces, third spaces (Lowe, 2014) or, in Winnicottian terms, potential spaces, within care homes, dividing lines exist between staff members and residents, and within each group, based on arbitrary categories (which nonetheless impact the lived experience, entering into individual psychic spaces) that prevent real engagement. An investigation of how categories of race, gender, and class intersect with the micro-interactions of daily relating in a dementia care context is vital in order to prevent entrenched power dynamics that fundamentally hinder intimacy and the sharing of human vulnerabilities.

I wish to turn momentarily to Jessica Benjamin (2018). Preoccupied by finding a way into relating beyond the power dynamics of doer and done-to, which arguably race and class categories feed into, Benjamin describes a process of mutuality which comes about through the development and subsequent engagement with thirdness. This is an important idea if we are to reflect on what a thinking space might offer an organisation such as Winston Grove or Whittinghall. To quote Benjamin (2018),

Rhythmic thirdness depends on co-creation, that is continuous mutual adjustment that persists through variation of patterns, which allows for acknowledgement of difference and deviation of both partners.

(p. 78–79)

Space to reflect upon the emotional labour – the power dynamics involved in human relating, the fear of causing further damage to objects already considered damaged – is certainly not advocated in *Living Well: A National Dementia Strategy*. As a result, many care organisations are ill-equipped to deal with the emotional cost of intimate human relating.

Dependency

Holding Time has been about the experience of dementia, and about the experience of working with people with dementia, in the care home site. It is also about our widespread anxiety about relating to dependency. Dependency in older people is particularly problematic because it reminds us of our own fear of decline; our fear that there will be no one there to catch us when we fall. It stirs up the nameless dread of fragmenting in isolation and returning to places we have possibly known but struggle to find words for. It feels all the more frightening because the political landscape that we know in the Western democracies is at present precarious, and the dependent are positioned as unlovable and insatiably needy. But, as Cooper & Lousada (2005, cited in Foster, 2010) point out, 'It is not dependency that is the problem, but fear and hatred of dependency which destroys the link to the source of support that may be the ground of our well-being' (p. 195). This source of support is arguably the relational. Our relationship with others, the huge potential for coming together when we share something of our fragility, is at stake. And our relationship with ourselves as human, with very real limits, too, also hangs in the balance.

The endless pursuit of living well, as found in the *National Dementia Strategy*, has not successfully embraced the ability to tolerate feelings of loss experienced in dementia, to acknowledge increasing disability, or to allow a trusting dependency to develop in relation to another person able to care. Is it alright to have bad, debilitating days? These are questions overlooked in the rhetoric. It seems possible that the idea of living well has been co-opted by the well, those who do not yet have dementia, because it allows us to pretend that dementia can be dressed up to look good in some way, that it is not quite as devastating as we think.

At the same time, neoliberal forms of government have also integrated notions of well-being into a network of discourses and practices that begin to support the dominant political ideology of our time. Living well, in neoliberal terms, can become a concept against which people, even the sickest and most incapacitated, can be judged. Incapacity, living unwell, in need of support – all this becomes shameful. In the (former) *Prime Minister's Challenge on Dementia* (2016) the 'wellness' discourse really takes hold with sections entitled, 'Living Well', 'Supporting Well', 'Training Well', 'Dying Well', 'Diagnosing Well'. There is no room for failing here.

There is a contradiction at the heart of the neoliberal agenda. It advocates autonomy and self-reliance on the one hand but also promotes an endless consumption. The neoliberal subject is invested in the idea that this process buys-in well-being, a kind of choosing that generates an 'appetite for appetite' (Phillips, 2005). Arguably this is about neediness, hunger, marketed and reframed as desire. This is perhaps the acceptable face of dependency, a dependency on the marketplace rather than on each other, through processes of noticing, play and meaning-making.

Of course, it is vital that we can make demands, have desires/wants, but the basis of our demands might need examining: what kinds of sustenance do we really need, particularly as our lives become more precarious?

The rational, self-possessed I, making choices and taking control, itself is mobilised in part to make policy more palatable. The notion of interiority is left unquestioned, assumed to belong entirely to the person with dementia or the family carer. This is a problematic area. Butler and Athanasiou (2013) suggest that possession is written into the basic structure of the neoliberal subject (I am in possession of myself, my rationality) but, as they argue, human subjects are always already dispossessed in the sense that their own minds, bodies, and experiences belong to and are given meaning through and with their relation to others.

For someone with dementia, a secondary dispossession takes place as their own mind becomes even further out of reach, and a need to trust increasingly another mind able to bear one's own emerges. Yet in current policy, the subject with dementia is implicitly conceived of as owning his or her mind continually throughout this wildly dispossessing journey. And those he or she relates to, the workforce, are seemingly untouched by him.

For me, the relational field as constituted in national policy within the UK presents difficulties because it doesn't make space for recognising the irrational, messy, uncertain, and confusing affective flows found in relating, or for the movement of dependencies between carers and people with dementia. The work of care is presented in a vocabulary that makes the experience more presentable, as if it is imperative that the difficulties be pushed out of view. Relationships shift in and out of asymmetries and symmetries, dialogues and monologues. Carers are both powerful and vulnerable in the same way that people with dementia are. Without reflecting upon the complex external dynamics and internal landscapes that lie between and within each party, the dangers are that relating becomes a fixed form and that organisational cultures close down to the wide range of experience involved in human encounter-events. It seems to me that meaningful encounter-events, which involve processes of self-fragilisation, between people sustain both the person with dementia in care homes and the person who cares for him. It seems vital that there is 'a re-evaluation of vulnerability as so much an essential part of human learning and living that far from evoking pity or contempt, it is respected as an ingredient in the glue of interpersonal solidarity'. (Froggett, 2002, p. 125)

Working with people with dementia and their carers allows me to conclude, then, something akin to Lynne Segal's claim that

> *Acknowledging the habitually disavowed mutual dependence necessary for sustaining the human condition, while querying our cultural obsession with notions of 'independence', just might help us to see that those most disparaged in the circuit of human interdependence, or largely abandoned within it, call into question the humanity in all of us.*
>
> (Segal, 2013, p. 37)

By hating dependency we also shame our infantile dependent self and shame ourselves as we age and move towards death. This is, quite simply, no way to go.

REFERENCES

Adams, T. and Gardiner, P. (2005) 'Communication and Interaction with Dementia Care Triads: Developing a Theory for Relationship-Centred Care.' In *Dementia*. 4(2), pp. 185–205

Alzheimer's Society (2017) 'Response to Spring Budget 2017 – the social care crisis is a dementia crisis.' Available at https://blog.alzheimers.org.uk/campaigns/response-to-spring-budget-2017/

Alzheimer's Society (n.d.) 'Financial Cost of Dementia.' Available at: https://www.alzheimers.org.uk/info/20091/what_we_think/146/financial_cost_of_dementia

Ainsworth, M. D. S., Blehar, M. C., Waters, E. & Wall, S. (1978) *Patterns of Attachment: A psychological study of the strange situation.* NJ: Lawrence Erlbaum

Appleby, J. (2013) 'Spending on Health and Social Care Over the Next 50 Years. Why Think Long-term?' The King's Fund. Available at https://www.kingsfund.org.uk/sites/files/kf/field/field_publication_file/Spending%20on%20health%20... %2050%20years%20low%20res%20for%20web.pdf

Armstrong, D. (2005a) *Organisation in the Mind: Psychoanalysis, Group Relations and Organisational Consultancy.* London: Karnac

Armstrong, D. (2005b) 'The "Institution in the Mind", Reflections on the Relation of Psychoanalysis to Work with Institutions. *The Human Nature Review.* http://human-nature.com/hraj/mind.html

Balfour, A. (2006) 'Thinking about the experience of dementia: The importance of the unconscious.' In *Journal of Social Work Practice.* 20(3), pp. 329–346

Baraitser, L. (2009) *Maternal Encounters: The Ethics of Interruption.* London: Routledge

BBConline (2014) Available at http://www.bbc.co.uk/news/uk-england-lancashire-25676842

BBConline (2014) Available at http://www.bbc.co.uk/news/uk-england-dorset-31417084

Benjamin, J. (2006) 'Recognition and Destruction: An Outline of Intersubjectivity.' In *Like Subjects, Love Objects: Essays on Recognition and Sexual Difference.* New Haven: Yale Press

Benjamin, J. (2007) 'Intersubjectivity, Thirdness, and Mutual Recognition'. A talk given at the Institute for Contemporary Psychoanalysis, Los Angeles

http://icpla.edu/wp-content/uploads/2013/03/Benjamin-J.-2007-ICP-
Presentation-Thirdness-present-send.pdf

Benjamin, J. (2010) 'Can We Recognise Each Other? Response to Donna
Orange.' In *International Journal of Psychoanalytic Self Psychology*, 5, pp. 244–256

Benjamin, J. (2018) *Beyond Doer and Done To: Recognition Theory, Intersubjectivity
and the Third*. London: Routledge

Bick, E. (1964) 'Notes on Infant Observation in Psychoanalytic Training.' In
Briggs, A. (ed.) (2002) *Surviving Space: Papers on Infant Observation*. London:
The Tavistock Clinic Series, pp. 37–55

Bion, WR. (1959) 'Attacks on Linking.' *International Journal of Psycho-Analysis*,
40(5–6), pp. 308–315

Bion, W. R. (1961) *Experiences in Groups*. London: Tavistock.

Bion, W.R. (1962a) *Learning from Experience*. Maryland: Maresfield Library

Bion, W. R. (1962b) 'The Psycho-Analytic Study of Thinking.' In *International
Journal of Psycho-Analysis*. 43, pp. 306–310

Boffey, D. (9 October 2016) 'Radical plan for old age as leak reveals care crisis.'
The Guardian. Available at https://www.theguardian.com/society/2016/
oct/09/social-care-crisis-looms-altmann

Bowlby, J. (1979) *The Making and Breaking of Affectional Bonds*. London:
Tavistock

Britton, R. (1989) 'The missing link: parental sexuality in the Oedipus
Complex.' In The Oedipus Complex Today, ed. J. Steiner, London: Karnac,
pp. 83–101

Britton, R. (1998) *Belief and Imagination*. London: The New Library of
Psychoanalysis

Britton, R. (2004) 'Subjectivity, Objectivity and Triangular Space.' In
Psychoanalytic Quarterly, 73, pp. 47–61

Browne, C. J. and Shlosberg, E. (2012) 'Attachment behaviours and parent
fixation in people with dementia: The role of cognitive functioning and pre-
morbid attachment style.' In *Aging & Mental Health*. London: Routledge

Butler, J. and Athanasiou, A. (2013) *Dispossession: The Performative in the Political*.
Cambridge: Polity Press

Butler, P. (18 October 2013) 'Jeremy Hunt: UK should adopt Asian culture of
caring for the elderly.' *The Guardian*. Available at https://www.theguardian.
com/politics/2013/oct/18/jeremy-hunt-uk-families-asia-elderly

Butler, P. (13 July 2016) 'Vulnerable adults at risk as councils face £1bn social
care shortfall.' *The Guardian*. Available at https://www.theguardian.com/
society/2016/jul/13/vulnerable-adult-social-care-risk-england-councils-face-
1bn-shortfall

Clark, D. (2018) 'Focus: a moment for dying and death?' In *Discover Society*, 6
February [Online]. Available at https://discoversociety.org/2018/02/06/focus-
a-moment-for-dying-and-death

Clarke, S. and Hoggett, P., eds. (2009) *Researching Beneath the Surface. Psycho-Social Research Methods in Practice.* London: Karnac

Clough, M. (2016) 'Shame: a risky emotion in dementia care.' In *Journal of Dementia Care,* 24(6), pp. 32–33

Cooper, A. and Lousada, J. (2005) *Borderline Welfare: Feeling and Fear of Feeling in Modern Welfare.* London: Karnac

Critchley, S. (1999) *Ethics–Politics–Subjectivity: Essays on Derrida, Levinas and Contemporary French Thought.* London: Verso

Crociani-Windland (2009) 'How to Live and Learn: learning, duration, and the virtual.' In Clarke, S. and Hoggett, P., (eds.) *Researching Beneath the Surface. Psycho-Social Research Methods in Practice.* London: Karnac, pp. 51–78

Crociani-Windland (2013) 'Old age and difficult life transitions: A Psychosocial Understanding.' *Psychoanalysis, Culture and Society.* 18(4), pp. 335–351

Dalal, F. (2002) *Race, Colour and the Processes of Racialization: New Perspectives from Group Analysis, Psychoanalysis and Sociology.* London: Routledge

Dartington, T. (2010) *Managing Vulnerability: The Underlying Dynamics of Systems of Care.* London: Karnac

Davenhill, R., Balfour, A., Rustin, M. and Pirozzolo, F.J. (2003) 'Looking into Later Life: psychodynamic observation and old age.' In *Psychoanalytic Psychotherapy,* 17(3), pp. 253–266

Davenhill, R. (2007) *Looking into Later Life: A Psychoanalytic Approach to Depression and Dementia in Old Age.* London: Karnac

Diamond, M. (2007) 'Organizational Change and The Analytic Third: Locating and Attending to Unconscious Psychodynamics.' In *Psychoanalysis, Culture and Society,* 12(2), pp.142–164

Dugan, E. (2014) 'Elderly Care Home Abuse.' *Independent.* Available at http://www.independent.co.uk/news/uk/home-news/shocking-footage-shows-elderly-residents-being-taunted-and-abused-at-essex-care-home-9303888.html

Ellis, M. and Astell, A. (2010) 'Communication and Personhood in Advanced Dementia.' *Healthcare Counselling & Psychotherapy Journal,* 10(3), pp. 32–35

Ettinger, B. (2006) 'Matrixial Trans-subjectivity.' In *Theory, Culture & Society,* 23(2–3), pp. 218–222

Ettinger, B. (2009) 'Fragilisation and Resistance.' In *Studies in the Maternal,* 1(2), pp. 1–31

Ettinger, B. (2010) '(M)Other Re-spect: Maternal Subjectivity, the Ready-made mother-monster and the Ethics of Respecting.' In *Studies in the Maternal,* 2(1), pp. 1–24

Frazer, S., Odeboyde, J. and Cleary, A. (2012) 'An interpretative phenomenological analysis: How older women who live alone with dementia make sense of their experiences.' In *Dementia,* 11(5), pp. 677–693

Freud, S. (1949) *An Outline of Psychoanalysis,* New York, W.W. Norton & Co. Inc., (1949), 109

Freud, S. (2005) *On Murder, Mourning and Melancholia*. London: Penguin Classics

Froggett, L. (2002) *Love, Hate and Welfare: Psychosocial Approaches to Policy and Practice*. Bristol: Policy Press

Froggett, L. and Briggs, S. (2012) 'Practice-near and practice-distant methods in human services research.' In *Journal of Research Practice*, 8(2), pp. 1–17

Gallagher, A. (22 February 2017) 'Let's tackle "careism" and give workers the respect they deserve.' Available at https://www.theguardian.com/social-care-network/social-life-blog/2017/feb/22/lets-tackle-careism-and-give-workers-the-respect-they-deserve

Hinshelwood, R.D. and Skogstad, W. (2000) *Observing Organisations*. London: Routledge

Hollway, W. (2011) 'Rereading Winnicott's "primary maternal preoccupation".' In *Feminism & Psychology*, 22(1), pp. 20–40

Hughes, G. and Lewis, G. (1998) *Unsettling Welfare: The Reconstruction of Social Policy*. London: Routledge

Hunter, S. (2015) *Power, Politics and the Emotions. Impossible Governance*. London: Routledge

Hutton, J., Bazalgette, J. and Reed, B. (1997) 'Organisation-in-the-mind.' In ed. J. Neumann, *Developing Organisational Consultancy*. London: Routledge

Jervis, L.L. (2001) 'The Pollution of Incontinence and the Dirty Work of Caregiving in a US Nursing Home.' In *Medical Anthropology Quarterly*, 15(1), pp. 84–99

Judah, Ben (2016) *This is London: Life and Death in the World City*. London: Picador

Keene, J. (2012) 'Reflections on the evolution of Independent psychoanalytic thought' in Williams, P., Keene, J. and Dermen, S. *Independent Psychoanalysis Today*. London: Karnac, pp3–47

Kitwood, T. (1997) *Dementia Reconsidered: The Person Comes First*. Buckingham: Open University Press

Kleijer B., van Marum R., Egberts A., Jansen P., Knol W. and Heerdink E. (2009) 'Risk of cerebrovascular events in elderly users of antipsychotics. In *Journal of Psychopharmacology*, 23, pp. 909–914

Klein, M. (1930 [1975]) 'The Importance of Symbol Formation in the Development of the Ego.' In *Love, Guilt and Reparation and Other Works 1921–1945*. New York: The Free Press. pp.219–232

Klein, M. (1937 [1975]) 'Love, Guilt and Reparation.' In *Love, Guilt and Reparation and Other Works 1921–1945*. New York: The Free Press. pp.306–343

Klein, M. (1940 [1975]) 'Mourning and its relation to Manic-Depressive States.' In *Love, Guilt and Reparation and Other Works 1921–1945*. New York: The Free Press. pp344–369

Klein, M. (1946 [1997]) 'Notes on Some Schizoid Mechanisms.' In *Envy and Gratitude and Other Works 1946–1963*. London: Vintage. pp. 1–24

Klein, M. (1952a [1997]) 'The Mutual Influences in the Development of Ego and Id.' In *Envy and Gratitude and Other Works 1946–1963*. London: Vintage. pp. 61–94

Klein, M. (1952b [1997]) 'Some Theoretical Conclusions Regarding the Emotional Life of the Infant.' in *Envy and Gratitude and Other Works 1946–1963*. London: Vintage. pp. 57–60

Klein, M (1952c [1997]) 'On Observing the Behaviour of Young Infants.' In *Envy and Gratitude and Other Works 1946–1963*. London: Vintage. pp. 94–122

Klein, M. (1957 [1997]) 'Envy and Gratitude.' In *Envy and Gratitude and Other Works 1946–1963*. London: Vintage. Pp. 176–235

Kontos, P. (2005) 'Embodied Selfhood in Alzheimer's Disease: Rethinking Person-Centred Care.' In *Dementia*, 4(4), pp. 553–570

Kontos, P., Miller, K.L., Colantonio, A. and Cott, C. (2014) 'Grief, Anger, and Relationality: The impact of a research based theatre intervention on emotion work practices in brain injury rehabilitation.' In *Evaluation Review*, 38(1), pp. 29–67

Kontos, P., Miller, K-L., and Kontos, A. (2017) 'Relational citizenship: Supporting embodied selfhood and relationality in dementia care.' In *Sociology of Health and Illness* (Special Issue: Ageing, Dementia and the Social Mind). DOI: 10.1111/1467-9566.12453

Kosofsky Sedgewick, E (2007) 'Melanie Klein and the Difference Affect Makes.' In *South Atlantic Quarterly*, 106(3), pp. 625–642

Kristeva, J. (1985) trans. by L. S. Roudiez 'Stabat Mater.' In *Poetics Today*, 6(1–2), pp. 133–152

Lacan J. (1956) Seminar on 'The Purloined Letter'. In Lacan, J. (2006) Écrits: The First Complete Edition in English (trans. by B. Fink). W.W. Norton & Co., New York

Lay, K. (2017) 'Social Care Cuts linked to 30,000 Excess Deaths.' In *The Times*. Available at https://www.thetimes.co.uk/article/social-care-cuts-linked-to-30-000-excess-deaths-mnwlq3l22

Layton, L. (2014) 'Some psychic effects of neoliberalism: Narcissism, disavowal, perversion.' In *Psychoanalysis, Culture and Society*, 19(2), pp. 161–178

Lewis, G. (2009) 'Animating hatreds: research encounters, organisational secrets, emotional truths.' In Ryan-Flood, Roisin and Gill, Rosalind eds. *Secrecy and Silence in the Research Process: Feminist Reflections. Transformations.* Abingdon: Routledge, pp. 211–227

Living Well: A National Dementia Strategy (Department of Health, 2009)

Lowe, F. ed. (2014) *Thinking Space: Promoting Thinking About Race, Culture, and Diversity in Psychotherapy and Beyond*. London: Karnac

Manthorpe, J. and Iliffe, S. (2016) 'The Dementia Strategy: time to change course.' In *Journal of Dementia Care*, 24(6), pp. 14–15

Matthews, F.E. et al. (2016) 'A two decade comparison of incidence of dementia in individuals aged 65 years and older from three geographical areas of England: results of the Cognitive Function Ageing Study I and II.' *Nature Communications*, DOI 10.1038/ncomms11398

Menzies Lyth, I. (1959) 'The Functions of Social Systems as a Defence Against Anxiety: A Report on a Study of the Nursing Service of a General Hospital', Human Relations 13: 95–121; reprinted in *Containing Anxiety in Institutions: Selected Essays, vol. 1*, Free Association Books, 1988, pp. 43–88

Merleau-Ponty, M. (1964) *The Primacy of Perception*. Chicago: Northwestern University Press

Miesen, B. M. L. (1993) 'Alzheimer's disease, the phenomenon of parent fixation and Bowlby attachment theory.' In *Internal Journal of Geriatric Psychiatry*, 8, p. 147–153

Miesen, B. M. L. (1999) *Dementia in close-up: Understanding and caring for people with dementia*. London: Routledge

Miller, L., Shuttleworth, J. and Rustin, M. (1989) *Closely Observed Infants*. London: Karnac

Millet, S. (2011) 'Self and embodiment: A bio-phenomenological approach to dementia.' In *Dementia*, 10(4), 509–522.

Nolan, M., Davies, S., Brown, J., Keady, J., and Nolan, J. (2004) 'Beyond Person-Centred Care: A New Vision for Gerontological Nursing.' In *Journal of Clinical Nursing*, 13(1), pp. 45–53.

Ogden, T. (1990a) 'The Mother, the Infant and the Matrix.' In *The Matrix of the Mind*, London: Maresfield Library, pp. 167–201

Ogden, T. (1990b) 'Internal Object Relations.' In *The Matrix of the Mind*, London: Maresfield Library, pp. 131–165

Osborne, H. and Duncan, P. (17 November 2016) 'Number of care workers on zero-hours contracts jumps from one to seven.' In *The Guardian*. Available at https://www.theguardian.com/uk-news/2016/nov/17/care-workers-zero-hours-contracts-unison-minimum-wage

Panorama: Nursing Homes Undercover (21 November 2016) BBC1

Phillips, A. (2005) *Going Sane: Maps of Happiness*. London: Fourth EstateSocial Care

Phillips, A. (2007) *Winnicott*. London: Penguin

Prime Minister's Challenge on Dementia (Department of Health, 2012)

Prime Minister's Challenge on Dementia 2020 (Department of Health, 2015)

Redman, P. (2009) 'Affect Revisited: Transference-countertransference and the unconscious dimensions of affective, felt and emotional experience.' *Subjectivity*, 25(1), pp. 51–68

Redman, P. (2016) 'Once more with feeling: What is the psychosocial anyway?' In *Journal of Psycho-Social Studies*, 9(1), pp. 73–93

Ryan, J. (2014) '"Class is in you": an exploration of some social class issues in psychotherapeutic work.' In Lowe, F. (ed.) *Thinking Space*. London: Karnac

Ryan, T., Nolan, M., Reid, D. and Enderby, P. (2008) 'Using the Senses Framework to achieve relationship-centred dementia care services.' In *Dementia*, 7(1), pp. 71–93

Sarton, M. (1983) *As We Are Now*. London: The Women's Press

Segal, L. (2013) *Out of Time: The Pleasures and Perils of Ageing*. London: Verso

Shuttleworth, J. (1989) 'Psychoanalytic Theory and Infant Development.' In *Closely Observed Infants*. London: Gerald Duckworth & Co. pp 22–51

Siddique, H. (14 November 2016) 'Dementia and Alzheimer's leading cause of death in England and Wales.' In *The Guardian*. Available at https://www.theguardian.com/society/2016/nov/14/dementia-and-alzheimers-leading-cause-of-death-england-and-wales

Sinason, V. 'The Man who was Losing his Brain.' In Sinason, V. (1992) *Mental Handicap and The Human Condition: New Approaches from the Tavistock*. London: Free Association Books

Sodha, S. (16 September 2016) 'Underfunded and Overstretched – the crisis in care for the elderly.' In *The Guardian*. Available at https://www.theguardian.com/society/2016/dec/10/care-for-elderly-crisis-how-to-improve-quality-of-life

Stephens, A., Cheston, R. and Gleeson, K. (2012) 'An exploration into the relationships people with dementia have with physical objects: An ethnographic study.' In *Dementia*, 12(6), pp 697–712

Taylor, D. (28 September 2015) 'Nigerian care workers to be deported after immigration raids.' In *The Guardian*. Available at https://www.theguardian.com/uk-news/2015/sep/28/nigerian-care-workers-to-be-deported-after-immigration-raids

Terry, P. (2003) *Working with the Elderly and their Carers: A Psychodynamic Approach*. London: Palgrave Macmillan

Terry, P. (2010) 'Dementia: A Psychodynamic Perspective.' In *Healthcare Counselling & Psychotherapy Journal*, 10(3), pp. 12–15

The Things between Us. Living Words: Anthology 1. Words of people experiencing dementia. (Edinburgh: Shoving Leopard, 2014)

University of Oxford (20 February 2017) '30,000 excess deaths linked to cuts in health and social care.' Available at http://www.ox.ac.uk/news/2017-02-20-30000-excess-deaths-2015-linked-cuts-health-and-social-care

Waddell, M. (2002) *Inside Lives: Psychoanalysis and the Growth of the Personality*. London, Karnac

Winnicott, D.W. (1946) eds. Caldwell, L. and Taylor Robinson, J. (2017) *The Collected Works of Donald Winnicott 1946–1951*. Oxford: Oxford University Press

Winnicott, D.W. (1953) 'Transitional objects and transitional phenomena.' In *International Journal of Psychoanalysis*, 34, pp. 89–97

Winnicott, D.W. (1958) 'Primary maternal preoccupation.' In *Collected papers: Through paediatrics to psychoanalysis*. London: Tavistock, pp. 300–305

Winnicott, D.W. (1960) 'The Theory of the Parent-Infant Relationship.' In *International Journal of Psycho-Analysis*, 41, pp. 585–595

Winnicott, D.W. (1962) 'On the Capacity to be Alone.' In *The Maturational Processes and the Facilitating Environment*. London: Hogarth Press, pp. 29–36

Winnicott, D.W. (2005 [1971]) *Playing and Reality*. London: Routledge Classics

World Health Organisation and Alzheimer's Disease International (2012) 'Dementia: a public health priority.' Available at http://www.who.int/mental_health/publications/dementia_report_2012/en/

Yalom, I.D. (2008) *Staring at the Sun: Overcoming the Dread of Death*. London: Piatkus Books